Health in Day Care: A Manual for Health Professionals

Author: Committee on Early Childhood,
Adoption and Dependent Care
American Academy of Pediatrics

Selma R. Deitch, M.D., Editor

American Academy of Pediatrics
P.O. Box 927, 141 Northwest Point Boulevard
Elk Grove Village, Illinois 60009

This document was supported in part by the Division of Maternal and Child Health and The Administration for Children, Youth and Families.

Library of Congress Catalog No. 87-70643

ISBN 0-910761-13-2

Single copy $25.00.
Quantity prices on request. Address all inquiries to:
American Academy of Pediatrics, P.O. Box 927, 141
Northwest Point Boulevard, Elk Grove Village, Illinois 60009

DEDICATION

To David Belais Friedman, M.D. (1916-1985) whose recognition of the health needs of children, of the receptivity of parents to help with parenting skills, of the value of day care of quality as a supplement to home care, and of the potential for the pediatrician to be helpful in providing useful consultation served to energize the Early Childhood, Adoption and Dependent Care Committee in the preparation of this manual.

FOREWORD

HISTORICAL PERSPECTIVE

The association of day care and health care is not new. When charitable agencies established the first day nurseries in New York and Boston in the midnineteenth century for "children of worthy working mothers," they certainly sought the counsel of physicians. As nursery school became a common experience for children from more affluent families in the early 1920s, the advice of pediatricians was sought by families in finding "good" schools. A pamphlet produced in the '20s by the Child Welfare League of America, entitled "Day Care, A Partnership of Three Professions," displayed on its cover a triangle with Health, Education, and Welfare forming the three sides.

In the early 1940s, under the leadership of Dr. Leona Baumgartner, a pediatrician who served as Commissioner of Health for the City of New York, a Division of Day Care, Day Camps, and Institutions was formed. This Division was responsible for licensing, counseling, and providing staff-parent education for daytime programs for children. Its staff consisted of early childhood educators and child welfare specialists who worked closely with public health nurses. Day care and health care became even more closely linked in New York when Dr. Harold Jacobziner, another pediatrician/public health physician, established health supervision clinics in some of the city's publicly supported day care centers in low-income areas.

The obligation of pediatricians to help in the development of sound day care programs became clearer after the establishment of the American Academy of Pediatrics (AAP) and its journal PEDIATRICS. Articles were published stressing the responsibility of pediatricians to take part in the day care field, and a statement to this effect, prepared by the Committee on Infant and Preschool Child, was printed in the AAP Newsletter of November 15, 1966.

Also in the '60s the Section of Maternal and Child Health (MCH) of the American Public Health Association took action that deepened the involvement of pediatricians in day care programs. An interdisciplinary committee set up by MCH with a pediatrician/public health physician as its chairman met under the sponsorship of the U.S. Children's Bureau in Washington. Dr. Katherine Bain, the Bureau's Chief of Research in Child Development, suggested that the MCH committee include representatives from the Child Welfare League and the American Academy of Pediatrics. The members of the AAP who attended the first two meetings of the committee, Drs. Samuel Karelitz, Edward Wakeman, Belle Dale Poole, and Patricia T. Schloesser, continued to work actively with the group as the MCH Committee established subcommittees on the care of infants, handicapped children, and the school-aged child. The MCH Committee carried out studies relating the extent of health involvement in child day care, and a pamphlet resulted, entitled "Day Care, with Focus on Health," edited by Laura Dittman and published by the Government Printing Office, as one of the Children's Bureau documents.

Federally sponsored programs for the supervision of children routinely involved day care. The Lanham Act financed child care centers during World War II that were open long hours, even overnight, to accommodate parents working on every shift. Funds were included for nurses and nutritionists acting as consultants. In 1965, Head Start began as a preschool summer child care program for poor children. The total needs of the child were addressed by adding medical, dental, and family components to this child care service.

Private resources have also been used to join day care and health care. Major contributions have been made to the understanding of health in day care by the Frank Porter Graham Child Development Center at the University of North Carolina in Chapel Hill. The Center's program, opened in 1966 and still in existence, has focused on childhood illness in the day care setting. It has carried out a number of significant studies that have resulted in new information regarding types, frequency, and management of infectious diseases in children.

By the 1970s health professionals, with pediatricians at the forefront, were organizing and articulating their advice for health maintenance in day care establishments. The Committee on Infant and Preschool Child of the American Academy of Pediatrics, under the chairmanship of Dr. Samuel

Karelitz, initiated the development of a statement on Standards for Day Care Centers for infants and children under three years of age. It was first published in 1971 and it was revised and expanded in 1973 under the direction of Dr. William B. Forsythe. The document was updated again by the committee in 1980 under the chairmanship of Dr. David B. Friedman. The present manual, which replaces the 1980 version, has been rewritten by the committee to include valuable advice from educators and social workers as well as pediatricians.

It is imperative to continue collaboration among all of the disciplines and individuals responsible for the health and welfare of children and their families. Wherever day care and health care services exist for families and children, physicians should continue to make their contribution to the promotion of the physical, social, and emotional well-being of the child.

Ann deHuff Peters, M.D.
La Jolla, California

ACKNOWLEDGMENTS

We wish to thank the many people who have offered us helpful suggestions, criticisms and corrections for the past two years as we prepared this manual. The following list includes names of those persons who have reviewed drafts or provided specific information. Surely, there are some persons whose names we have missed and for this we apologize.

Susan S. Aronson	Jeanne M. Hunzeker
Glen S. Bartlett	Vince L. Hutchins
Robert F. Biehl	Richard B. Kearsley
Helen Blank	Earline Kendall
Philip A. Brunell	Stanley I. Levine
Bettye Caldwell	Alvin M. Mauer
Robert W. Chamberlin, Jr.	Gwen Morgan
Albert Chang	Linda J. Morgan
Thomas Coleman	Shirley Norris
Lucy S. Crain	Ann DeHuff Peters
Laura L. Dittmann	Stanley A. Plotkin
Paul G. Dyment	June Solnit Sale
Antoinette P. Eaton	Joe M. Sanders, Jr.
Judith L. Evans	Daniel W. Shea
David B. Friedman (deceased)	Patricia T. Schloesser
Geraldine Norris Funke	Phyllis E. Stubbs
Bruce M. Gach	Bernice Weissbourd
Albert L. Gaskins	Kathryn Young
G. Scott Giebink	Joseph R. Zanga
Lindsey K. Grossman	Edward Zigler
Margie Hale	Barry S. Zuckerman
H. James Holroyd	

Certain individuals deserve special mention for their contributions to particular chapters and their extensive help throughout the project. Linda Morgan added significantly to Chapter I and assisted in choosing the information to be included in the rest of the manual and the order in which it should be presented; Kay Lewis, the new liaison representative to our Committee, responded willingly to the request for aid with the form and substance of Chapter III; Sue Aronson, the Committee's consultant on day care, provided important material for Chapters VI and VII as well as constant support, encouragement, and prompt response in times of crisis. Finally, we remember with gratitude not only his work on Chapter VIII but also the empathy, gentle guidance and words of wisdom generously provided by the late David B. Friedman.

The continuity of the text and its uniformity of style were produced by our copy editor, Barbara J. Stahl. The many drafts were typed, ordered, and corrected with patience by Stacey Droboty and Debbie Shapiro.

Selma R. Deitch, M.D.
Editor

INTRODUCTION

This manual is addressed primarily to physicians, especially community pediatricians, who are increasingly called upon for advice concerning the health maintenance of children in day care facilities. Administrators and staff of these facilities, as well as parents of children served by them, frequently have questions about health issues that can be answered authoritatively only by professional health care personnel. The material presented in the manual will be useful not only to physicians faced with these questions, but also to epidemiologists, sanitarians, and public health and community nurses. Individuals not trained in health care, but who are responsible for health-related aspects of child care programs, may also find this manual helpful, particularly with the assistance of a health consultant.

Since the American Academy of Pediatrics published *Standards for Day Care Centers* in 1971, day care programs have expanded significantly. The central office of the Academy and members of its Committee on Early Childhood, Adoption, and Dependent Care have received requests from diverse groups for more information than the 1971 publication provided. Practicing physicians, health departments, parent support groups, and newspaper and magazine feature writers pose questions about checklists for assessing the quality of day care, the management of a specific communicable disease, alternative care for the sick child, policies for the child with special needs, and the health considerations of day care for infants. This manual supplies answers to these and other questions on health-related topics for the current time. More specific information related to health topics covered here may be found in other publications of the American Academy of Pediatrics, e.g., *The Pediatric Nutrition Handbook*. The adaptation of the general information presented requires collaboration between health and day care professionals with an interest in the same day care programs.

The AAP recognizes the contributions that other human service groups have made to the literature on day care programs and facilities. The Child Welfare League of America (CWLA) issued a revised version of its Standards for Day Care Service in 1984, and, also in 1984, the National Association for the Education of Young Children (NAEYC) published the Accreditation Criteria and Procedures of the National Academy of Early Childhood Programs. These documents make valuable recommendations to administrators, educators, social workers, and health workers regarding staff qualifications, physical site, curriculum, training of personnel, program administration, and the role of parents. Because the subject matter in these areas is treated with an expertise often not possessed by the physician asked for advice about day care, the readers of this manual are urged to use these other sources.

The chapters that follow in this book present the child care setting; the interplay of child, family, and professionals therein; and the health, growth, and developmental factors that require the physician's attention. In the Foreword, Dr. Ann deHuff Peters described the long history of collaboration between pediatricians and child care providers. To bring the reader up-to-date concerning the commitment of the AAP, the Academy's statement "The Pediatrician's Role in Promoting the Health of a Patient in Day Care" is reprinted from the July 1984 issue of PEDIATRICS (see Appendix I.1).

The first four chapters supply information about day care necessary for the physician who is asked to recommend measures for health promotion in care facilities. Just as doctors have to assess the child for whom they would prescribe treatment, so they have to know the setting for which they suggest health maintenance procedures. The first chapter traces the positive effect of a nurturing environment upon the development of the infant and child from the residential infant care provided at the turn of the century to the well-run modern day care programs that supplement care at home. Following that overview, Chapter II sets forth precise suggestions for program components that advance the health of the child. Attention is given to the unique characteristics of the child and the modification of environmental factors such as nutrition that will enhance growth and development. A strong plea is made to support parents' involvement in the day care choice and program. The child with special needs is covered in Chapter III. The text elucidates the role of the pediatrician in advocating day care adapted to serve this child effectively and discusses a variety of settings in which children with different disabilities can be accommodated. The fourth chapter in this section addresses the issue of child abuse, a phenomenon reported with increasing frequency. It analyzes thoroughly its prevention, recognition, and management.

The remaining chapters treat health care provision and management specifically. Chapter V describes measures that retard the spread of contagious diseases in day care facilities and makes practical suggestions for the prevention of infection. The subject is crucial because questions related to infections are those most frequently asked of the health professional by the child care providers. The sixth chapter reviews factors that increase the risk of injury to children in the day care setting. Rules are provided for the maintenance of a safe environment and advice is given for handling injuries that do occur. Besides organizing material for the physician, these two chapters will be an excellent resource for child care administrators responsible for training staff members and developing policies regarding health and safety.

Chapters VII, VIII, and IX have been included in the manual to supply information that will render health professionals more effective as consultants. It is the Committee's hope that physicians and other workers in the health care field will be encouraged to make themselves more accessible to child care providers. Now that the number of children cared for outside the home is growing, it is time for physicians who have occasionally given advice over the telephone to involve themselves more intimately in the day care setting. Their help is needed, for instance, by day care providers training staff members in health measures. Chapter VII includes useful comments on the scheduling of such training, subjects to be taught, and teaching methods that work.

The eighth chapter, "The Health Professional as a Health Consultant to Day Care Programs," is a revision of a chapter that appeared in the 1971 AAP day care manual. Written in the form of a guide for the pediatrician who is called upon or has volunteered to serve as a consultant, this section offers general instructions for advising and summarizes some of the material dealt with in greater detail elsewhere. Health professionals acting as consultants must be familiar with regulations for day care in their own communities, whether they emanate from the municipal, state, or federal level. The final chapter emphasizes this point and describes ways in which health care providers can help to change policies governing health-related agencies. Health advisory councils are described and health professionals are urged to participate in their development and activities.

The Appendices provide sample letters, forms, and checklists that will save readers the labor of creating their own. The Committee intends this manual to serve as a reference on the several topics it covers, and so has made each chapter comprehensive despite the risk of repeating some information. If the purpose of the Committee is fulfilled, physicians and other health professionals should be able to increase their contribution to day care of high quality for the young children who are of concern to all of us.

Selma R. Deitch, M.D., Editor
For The Committee on Early Childhood Development, Adoption, and Dependent Care
American Academy of Pediatrics

DEFINITION OF DAY CARE

Day care means the care, supervision, and guidance of a child or children, unaccompanied by parent or other legal custodian, on a regular basis, for periods of less than 24 hours. Included in the definition are the following examples:

- Regular babysitters in the child's home.
- Family day care (care of six* or fewer children in the caregiver's home).
- Share care (care of a few children of several families in the home of one of the parents).
- Group homes (six to twelve* children in a residence, with more than one caregiver to meet ratio requirements).
- Day care centers, either part-day or full-day, including Head Start, nursery schools, full-day centers, centers that care for infants, centers that care for preschool children, centers that care for school-aged children before and after school and during vacations, centers that care for children of different ages, and centers that care for children with special needs.
- Child care that meets the needs of parents who work nights or require supervised child care for parts of a day (e.g., night care or drop-in care).

Terms used in designating special forms and components of day care are defined in Appendix I.2.

For the purposes of this manual, we are not including in the term day care any of the arrangements that parents are able to make for the care of their children within the resources of the family and its very close friends. About half of working parents are able to make such arrangements. Examples of care excluded from the definition are:

- A parent on maternity or paternity leave from work
- A parent working at home
- Parents staggering their work hours so that someone will be at home at all times
- An older sibling caring for a younger one

---

*The numbers used in defining this category of care will vary from state to state.

- A relative or very close friend caring for the child in the child's own home
- A relative or very close friend caring for the child in the relative's home
- The child caring for himself or herself (latch-key child)

CONTENTS

Chapter 1

PROMOTION OF DEVELOPMENT IN THE OUT-OF-HOME CHILD CARE SETTING

1.1 Introduction

The term day care is used to describe any child care super-vision provided out of the home by persons other than the parents or in the home by a nonfamily member. The use of such care for children has become increasingly widespread in many countries, including the United States. However, the care of children even part time outside the nuclear family has raised many concerns. The implications of such day care for children's health, emotional state, and psychological de-velopment continue to be controversial. When consulted about the advisability of day care, the physician frequently feels uncomfortable rendering a professional opinion. Yet the physician is often regarded by parents as the likely source of such an expert opinion.

The impact of child-rearing settings on children has been under investigation since the turn of the century. Early studies focused on mortality, but more recently the complex issue of morbidity has been addressed. The results of these investigations provide reassuring information about alterna-tive child-rearing settings which are becoming increasingly necessary in our society. This chapter will provide a brief review of some of the studies, a description of the need for day care and a discussion of the physician's role in assuring good day care services for children.

1.2 Studies of Child Rearing

In 1908 Dr. Harry Dwight Chapin, a pediatrician in New York, described a marked decrease in mortality of infants who were moved from institutions to foster homes with close medical and nursing supervision. In some institutions at the time infant mortality approached 100%. Placement in a foster home reduced mortality significantly.[1]

Despite presentation of these findings in national pediatric journals and at meetings, many infants continued to be sent to orphanages. The persistent use of orphanages and similar institutions resulted in part from the authorities' efforts to prevent the entrance into adoptive or foster homes of persons who, in the early 1900s, were referred to as "mentally defective" or "feeble-minded." Typically, infants were tested between one and two years of age to determine mental ability. Since prevailing developmental theory held that ability was fixed, being determined by heredity and unaffected by environment, "retarded" infants were expected to become "retarded" children and adults, continuously in need of supervision. In countless cases, retention of these infants in institutions actually caused retarded functioning.

In the 1930s a serendipitous observation by Skeels, a psychologist in Iowa, provided the basis for a classic experiment demonstrating the marked effect of environment on development. Skeels had tested and certified that a 13- and a 16-month-old were functioning at an "imbecile level of mental retardation." The children were accordingly transferred from the nursery orphanage to an institution for the feeble-minded. Six months later, Skeels came across these children on the ward of the institution. Much to his surprise, these children appeared to be functioning normally. He re-tested them and found changes of 31 and 52 IQ points. These astonishing results led him to undertake a rather unusual experiment. As he stated, he arranged the "transfer of mentally retarded children in the orphanage nursery, one to two years of age, to an institution for feeble-minded in order to make them normal." All the transferred children showed gains on IQ tests ($\bar{x}$ = +27.5, range = 7 to 49 points) and in their general level of performance. Conversely, a contrast group who remained at the orphanage showed a progressive decrease in performance on IQ tests ($\bar{x}$ = −26.2, range = +2 to −45 points).[2] Analysis of the transferred infants' environment indicated that the staff and inmates "adopted" these infants, providing stimulation and nurturance which was absent at the orphanage. The infants were subsequently placed in adoptive homes, and follow-up into adulthood indicated that they continued to do well.[3]

This landmark study demonstrated that environment, particularly one with extreme stimulus deprivation, had a marked effect on child development. Furthermore, the study showed that it was not the institutional setting *per se*, but the degree of stimulation and caregiver responsiveness that was critical to successful development during the first few years of life.

Like Chapin's 1908 work, Skeels' study was largely ignored for some time. The negative impact of a poor environment on children's physical well-being identified by Chapin and by Skeels was rediscovered in the 1940s and '50s. Maternal deprivation was presented as a major causative factor in nonorganic failure to thrive. Singling out this environmental component, Spitz identified the absence of mother love as the cause of the physical and psychoemotional syndrome of retardation that he termed anaclitic depression. The key role played by environment on the growth of infants was firmly established.

However, the exact nature of the optimal environment needed further delineation. Theory of the 1940s and '50s postulated that only mothers in the home could foster normal development. The World Health Organization's Expert Committee led by Bowlby in 1951 stated that day nurseries and creches inevitably caused "permanent damage to the emotional health of a future generation."[4]

Margaret Mead, addressing the American Psychiatric Association, expressed a contrary point of view:

This, as Hilde Bruch has cogently pointed out, is a new and subtle form of antifeminism in which men—under the guise of exalting the importance of maternity—are tying women more tightly to their children. . . .anthropological evidence gives no support at present to the value of such an accentuation of the tie between mother and child.[5]

The controversy about the importance of the mother's presence persists, but as Rutter has pointed out, earlier studies failed to make the key distinction between maternal deprivation and general environmental deprivation, which frequently coincide. Children reared in various settings with one or a few consistent caregivers other than the mother, who provide adequate stimulation, show no untoward effects—psychologically, socially, or emotionally.[6,7,8]

Later studies clearly support the observations of Skeels and Dye: adequate stimulation and nurturance provided by a stable group of caregivers are crucial for normal development during the first years of life. This point is borne out by analyses of children in Head Start, the extensively studied preschool day care program launched in 1965. Initial reports were disappointing in that the gains made by Head Start children in cognitive performance, as measured by IQ tests, had disappeared after school entry. This was touted as evidence for the futility of early education for disadvantaged children. The theorists who consider genetically determined inferiority an important factor in the disadvantaged, predominantly black population cite these early studies as proof of their premise. However, continued investigation has led to significantly different results and conclusions.

Long-term studies have documented a marked difference in the need for remedial services during the school years on the part of children who did and did not attend Head Start. Children involved in Head Start programs of high quality failed promotion less frequently, needed fewer special education classes, and completed high school in greater numbers than children not enrolled in the experimental preschool programs. Even more important, as adults they achieved a higher rate of employment and held better-paying jobs. The cost/benefit ratio of Head Start calculated only on the basis of decreased need of special education services demonstrated that this program was extraordinarily economical.[9,10]

Even more impressive gains have been found at the Frank Porter Graham Development Center in Chapel Hill, North Carolina. An experimental study in which infants from disadvantaged homes were placed in full-time day care until school age has shown that these children functioned in school at a level far superior to those in a matched group not given day care. A startling by-product of this intervention was that the parents of children in the day care group went on to obtain further education and better jobs. Thus, the parents improved their socio-economic status markedly, even though there had not been any specific parent-training component in the day care program.[11,12]

The studies cited here and others like them have not ended the argument between the proponents for heredity and those for environment as the major determinant of human development. The classic controversy continues, providing a dialectic that influences issues relevant to child care.[13] Whatever the balance between genetic endowment and environmental influences, the fact remains that only the environment can be manipulated; changing it has resulted in significant improvement of performance. Currently, we have sufficient knowledge to define elements of the environment that will affect the quality of care either in the home or in a day care setting. The requirement of day care for children of working mothers need not be deplored as a necessity that inevitably compromises normal development. In fact, for children from marginal home situations, day care may enhance performance and abilities.[14,15,16]

1.3 Need for Day Care

In the United States the supply of child care lags so far behind the demand that more than one child in six under 13 years old, including many preschoolers, may lack adult supervision when a parent is away. The need for infant care is a problem in almost every American community, as is the scarcity of after-school programs for young children who are sometimes left waiting up to four hours a day in empty homes, in school yards, or on neighborhood streets, while parents work. San Francisco's Information and Referral Services reported that in the final quarter of 1984, over 55% of requests were for care for infants from birth to two, with 40% of these for infants under seven months. Parents who cannot afford the full fee for infant care may find that there is an 18 to 24-month wait for a place in a subsidized program. The number of working women with children has increased dramatically in the years following World War II. Only 29% of women with children under age 18 were in the labor force in 1947; in contrast, 60% of these women were employed in 1982, a three-fold increase in about 30 years. As more and more parents of young children work, child care needs will become an even greater problem.

The following statistics provide further indication of this need:

- Almost 47% of married mothers whose youngest child is under one year of age are in the labor force, a 95% increase since 1970.
- Among married mothers with children whose youngest child is two years of age, 53.5% are in the labor force, a 75% increase since 1970.
- Almost 58% of married mothers whose youngest child is under age three are in the labor force.
- Of all mothers married and unmarried, more than 52% with children under age six are in the labor force.
- Over nine million children under age six have mothers in the labor force.
- Over 15 million children under age 13 have mothers in the labor force.
- Most employed mothers—71% in March 1984—work full-time. Even when their youngest child is under three, about 65% of employed mothers are full-time workers.[17]

Every mother who works has to face and solve the problem of child care. There are particular situations, however, where the parent or the child is at special risk unless adequate day care service is available. Without such service, for instance, adolescent parents cannot return to school to complete their education. Every year 523,000 babies are born to teenage girls; if these young women have to drop out of school, they reduce their chances of getting a job that would ultimately make them self-supporting. Abused and neglected children constitute another group for which child care is a priority. Parents of handicapped children are also desperately in need of care facilities. The 500,000 handicapped children under age 6 and the 3.7 million of school age commonly have special requirements. In many cases, the best way to reduce family stress and protect the children from harm is to separate the children from the parents for all or part of the day.

We know that nearly all mothers are working because they need the income and most need assistance to obtain quality child care. In 1983, two thirds of all women in the labor force were single, widowed, divorced, or had husbands who earned less than $15,000.

Increasing the availability of child care programs is only half the battle. The other half is financing them. The parents who need day care service most are frequently those least able to pay for it. A mother who heads a single-parent household often subsists near or below the poverty line. In 1982, the average single mother with children at home earned only $8,951. In most communities, she would have had to pay almost one third of her income to purchase center-based child care. This is three times more than the 10% of the budget considered reasonable for child care expenses. Despite their limited resources, single mothers are compelled to seek places to leave their children while they work. The Child Care Information and Referral Service in Cleveland received 30% of its calls in 1984 from women in this category; and 70% earned less than $10,500 annually. These working mothers need help in meeting their child care costs.

The availability of financial assistance for day care could make a difference in the lives of a significant number of the nation's children. Currently, over 12 million children under 18 years of age, or one in five, live in a single-parent family headed by the mother. By 1990, the ratio is expected to be one in four, double that of 1970. Already, half of all black children live with their mothers only. Many of the children who have two working parents should be included among those who would benefit: 25% of married women who work outside the home have husbands who earn less than $10,000. Since more than half the women who are employed also make less than $10,000, the combined income of husband and wife does not always guarantee ability to pay what day care may require.

The lack of child care programs and the paucity of financial assistance to pay for them are major factors in keeping women and children in poverty. A recent Census Bureau survey asked the majority of mothers who are not in the labor force whether they would work if child care were available at a reasonable cost. Forty-five percent of the single mothers in the survey replied affirmatively, as did 36% of all mothers (single parents and those in two-parent households) with family incomes under $15,000. Obviously, there are good arguments for supporting child care initiatives.[18]

1.4 The Physician's Role

Physicians have a strong interest in day care. Their key role in reducing child mortality in the past and their present involvement in limiting childhood morbidity leads them to recognize the child care setting as an important factor in the healthy functioning of children. Because more and more infants, preschoolers, and early school-aged children are spending a large part of each day in out-of-home care centers, physicians find themselves calculating the effect of nonparental caregivers as well as family members on the maturing child. To assure the well-being of a child, the physician can encourage families to look for, and even help them to find a care program with a well-trained, responsive staff, and clean, safe quarters.

Physicians can help day care administrators and staff members as well as parents by sharing their knowledge of the unique characteristics of a child. Planners and caregivers in out-of-home facilities, like parents, have to be able to recognize each child's level of functioning, anticipate emerging skills, and design approaches that enable the child to achieve specific goals at various stages of development. By promoting communication among the people who care for a child in and out of the home, the physician can help assure that the child's special needs will be addressed consistently. To perform this function effectively, the physician has to be well-informed about day care and willing to allot the time required to provide consultative services to families and day care staff.

Because the public has great respect for their judgment and expertise, physicians can be powerful advocates for day care of good quality in their communities. Advocacy, however, draws the doctor into the intertwined and unresolved issues associated with day care everywhere. Quality, caregiver wages, and the affordability of the service are interlinked; increasing the size of the staff or offering higher salaries to attract desirable workers and competent administrators raises operating cost and the quality of care improves, but it becomes unaffordable for more people. Since reductions in staff and reductions in the wages of child care providers, who are notoriously underpaid in the first place, are directly related to loss of quality in a program, the best solution is often public or private subsidy. Physicians can voice support for the legislation of tax credits for day care expenses or the establishment of scholarships or any mechanism they think appropriate to solve the financial problem.

Finally, physicians can determine the features of a child care program that encourages wholesome child development and communicate them to parents and the public at large. Doubtless, every physician will make his or her own assessment of what is necessary for optimal care, but the following list presents a set of basic priorities. A good care program should:

- Provide a safe, secure setting for children whose parents must be away from them for part of the 24-hour day.
- Utilize as caregivers persons of good character who are properly trained and naturally warm and responsive to children.
- Promote sound health and the development of physical abilities.
- Offer a stimulating environment where children will be able to master cognitive and communicative skills.
- Encourage children to develop at their own rate.
- Nurture the children's self-confidence, curiosity, creativity, and self-discipline.
- Stimulate children to ask questions, solve problems, make decisions, engage in activities, and explore and experiment with their environment.
- Foster the children's skill in social relationships, their sense of self-esteem, and an understanding of the common human dignity that underlies racial and ethnic differences.
- Provide guidance for the children and help for parents in improving their child-raising skills.
- Promote cooperation among parents, caregivers, public and private schools, and the community.[19]

Physicians, community nurses, social workers, educators, and others who touch the lives of children can, if they inform themselves about day care and work together, bring about a transformation in the field of child supervision and development.

References

1. Chapin HD: A *plan* of dealing with atrophic infants and children. *Arch Ped* 1908;25:491-496
2. Skeels HM, Dye HB: A study of the effects of differential stimulation on mentally retarded children. *Am J Ment Defic* 1939; 44:114-136
3. Skeels HM: Adult status of children with contrasting early life

experiences, in *Monographs of the Society for Research in Child Development*, Vol. 31 (3, Serial No. 105), 1966

4. World Health Organization *Expert Committee On Mental Health, Report Of The Second Session*, Technical Report Series, No. 31 Geneva, World Health Organization, 1951. Quoted in Clarke AM, Clarke ADB: The formative years? in Clarke AM, Clarke ADB: *Early Experience: Myth and Evidence*. New York, The Free Press, 1979, p 23

5. Mead M: Some theoretical considerations on the problem of mother-child separation. *Am J Orthopsychiatry* 1954;24:471-483

6. Rutter M: Maternal deprivation, 1972-1978: New findings, new concepts, new approaches. *Child Dev* 1979;50:283-285

7. Rutter M: *Maternal Deprivation Reassessed*. Hammondsworth, Middlesex, Penguin, 1972

8. Rutter M: Separation experiences: A new look at an old topic. *J Pediatr* 1979;95:147-154

9. Lazar I, Darlington R: Lasting effects of early education: A report from the Consortium for Longitudinal Studies. Monographs of the Society for Researching Child Development. Vol. 47, (Nos 2-3), 1982

10. Zigler E, Valentine J, (ed): *Project Head Start. A Legacy of the War on Poverty*. New York, The Free Press, 1979

11. Ramey CT, MacPhee D, Yeates KO: Preventing developmental retardation. Paper presented at the Sixth Vermont Conference on the Primary Prevention of Psychopathology. Burlington, VT, June 1980

12. Ramey CT, Farran DC, Campbell FA: Predicting IQ from mother-infant interactions. *Child Dev* 1979;50:804-814

13. Gould SJ: *The Mismeasure of Man*. New York, WW Norton and Company, 1981

14. Guinagh BJ, Jester RE: Long term effects of infant stimulation programs, in Camp BW, (ed): *Advances in Behavioral Pediatrics*, Vol 2. Greenwich, CT, JAI Press, 1981

15. Belsky J, Steinberg LD: The effects of day care: A critical review. *Child Dev* 1978;49:929-949

16. Kagan J, Kearsley RB, Zelazo PR: *Infancy. Its Place in Human Development*, Cambridge, MA, Harvard University Press, 1980

17. Hayghe H: Working mothers reach a record number in 1984. Research summaries in *Monthly Labor Review*, Office of Employment and Unemployment Statistics. U.S. Bureau of Labor Statistics. Washington, DC, December 1984, pp 31-34

18. Blank H: Overview of Child Care, Austin, Texas. Children's Defense Fund, Washington, DC, February 1985 (unpublished presentation)

19. Child Welfare Services: *Standards for Day Care Services*, revised. New York, Child Welfare League of America, Inc, 1984

Chapter 2

KEEPING THE CHILD HEALTHY IN THE DAY CARE SETTING

2.1 Introduction

Protection from environmental hazards, prevention of illness, and promotion of well-being are important in the day care setting just as they are in the home setting. As physicians and other providers of health care recognize, good intentions are not in themselves sufficient to assure the health and happiness of children in either place. The day care program, however informal the setting, should make adaptations that promote the children's physical, communicative, social and cognitive development. If the methods used are successful, they will reduce the incidence of destructive, resistive, purposeless behaviors, high activity levels, and poor dietary habits (the "new morbidities") in the population served.[1]

This chapter describes and recommends practices that help to assure the health of the children collectively and that provide a good experience for each child. No attempt is made to cover every aspect of the day care operation.

2.2 Factors Supportive of the Health of Children in Child Care Programs

2.2.A Personnel

The day care staff is immediately responsible for the ambiance of the care center: a child's ability to adjust and flourish in a program is in great part dependent upon his reaction to and feelings about the people who are in charge. It is not enough, however, to choose as staff members affectionate individuals whom the children like. A warm and affectionate nature and a love for children are necessary in a caregiver, but the staff member also has to have the ability to do things necessary to safeguard children and enhance their development. Staff members should have learned, if not through special training, at least by long experience, to recognize children's needs as they change from stage to stage and indeed sometimes from hour to hour. Besides being sensitive in their reactions, caregivers have to be creative: it requires imagination to plan and initiate activities and to respond on the spur of the moment to situations as they arise. Patience is another requirement; no matter how tired they are or how exasperating a child may be, staff people must be able to continue calm, consistent management of the child's behavior and avoid disturbance in the group. They should have the natural leadership that makes the job of controlling the group easier.

Ideally, caregivers should be skilled in verbal communication. Since the future development of the children depends to no small degree on their command of language, the opportunity should not be lost to encourage preschool children to express their thoughts verbally. Articulate caregivers should talk with young children and give them an opportunity to use language. Communication should start with the response to and encouragement of soft infant sounds. Caregivers should be talking to the young infants as they feed, change, and cuddle them. Naming objects and singing rhymes are appreciated by the midinfancy child, and imitation begins. Vocabulary soon explodes and verbal expression begins to accompany play. Richness of language increases as it is nurtured by verbal interaction of the child with adults and peers. It is desirable that a member of the staff be able to communicate in the primary language of the children.

Administrators screening prospective staff members should look, of course, for nurturing persons with mature judgment and the ability to understand and carry out the procedures that ensure safety and sanitation. Finally, individuals who are entrusted with the care of children should be demonstrably in good physical and mental health.

In a group setting caregivers work not only individually but as a team. Under the direction of the program administrator, staff members sharpen their own skills and improve their interaction. It follows that the stability of the staff will affect the care and confidence of the children: children benefit from continuity of personnel, not having to adjust to the loss—or repeated loss—of persons to whom they are attached. When a member of the staff is going to depart, it is advisable to prepare the children ahead of time for the transition to another adult. The sudden disappearance of a familiar friend and caregiver can be upsetting to a child of any age. Changing the composition of the group with the resultant loss of a companion can also be upsetting, particularly to the preschooler and early school-aged child.

Even a stable staff of competent caregivers cannot make up for an inadequate adult/child ratio. The staff must be large enough so that its members can take time to relate to the children as individuals and in a group. The optimal number of caregivers will vary with the age and social maturity of children in the program. Day care licensing requirements state minimum adult/child ratios: they reflect the fact that infants and children with special needs require more adult attention, whereas older children can function well in large groups for parts of the day. The proper ratio is a practical matter. There must be enough adults present to

• Supervise other members of the group of children when full attention of one adult is required by a single child
• Feed infants individually
• Supervise washing or wash children's hands before meals and after use of the toilet
• Help small children with outer clothes
• Provide for the safety of children in transport vehicles
• Promote child development rather than simply keep order
• Evacuate all children from a facility in an emergency

2.2.B The Physical Setting

Good child care can be achieved in a variety of physical settings, but there are some specifications that all facilities should meet. Some relate to safety directly—and these are usually outlined in local building and fire department regulations—but others affect the well-being of children in more subtle ways.

Space is important. Crowding, besides making contagion more difficult to control, has a negative effect on children's activities and states of mind. There is no consensus on the exact amount of floor space required per child, and no scientific basis for a particular figure exists. State regulations frequently cite as a minimum 35 square feet per child of clear floor area, exclusive of hallways and toilet areas. However, Prescott recommends 50 square feet.[2] Outdoor space should be even larger: to allow running and milling about, state regulations often stipulate 75 square feet per child using the space at one time.

The indoor site should be well lit. Children should be in the proper temperature indoors and out. Optimal room temperature is 68° to 72°. It should be measured at a level where children's activity takes place. This will vary according to the age of the children and the activity in which they are engaged. Regional climatic conditions should also be considered. Air conditioning may be necessary in climates where cooling is of equal importance to heating. Comfort of children and staff is the major objective of climate control.[2] When children go outdoors, it is essential that their clothing be appropriate for the weather. When weather conditions become extreme, outdoor play is best curtailed.

The use and ordering of indoor space should be carefully considered. Besides arranging activity areas conveniently in relation to one another and to entrances and exits, planners should allow places that individual children can identify as their own. Whether a crib, a mat, a cubby, or a quiet corner, the child's designated area should provide a sense of privacy and possession. In one or more of these places, the child should have access to safe toys to play with. Having a sufficient number of such toys available allows the child freedom of choice and reduces the need to wait or fight for what he or she wants.

2.2.C Schedule of Activities

The schedule of activities is determined largely by the physical, social, and cognitive needs of the children and is, of necessity, geared to the group. There should be sufficient flexibility, however, to accommodate the temperament of individuals. Sometimes the need for such accommodation is temporary: a child new to the program may be slow to engage in ongoing activities and cautious in relating to other children and adults. Altering his schedule initially may have a bearing upon his successful introduction to day care.

2.2.D Rest

For the young infant it is important that the adult provide favorable conditions for sleep. These include being dry, well-fed, and comfortable. Also conducive to sleep are a consistent caregiver and a routine for comforting, a reasonably quiet place, and a regularity in time for rest.[3] It is generally accepted that most preschool children in all-day care will benefit from scheduled periods of rest. Suiting the rest requirements and resting behavior of numerous children is not easily done, particularly in a setting with a range of age from infancy through preschool years. Some three-year-olds have given up naps, whereas some five-year-olds still take them. Some children are used to napping in the late morning rather than early afternoon when most centers schedule the quiet period. There are children who rest without sleeping and others who sleep but who have props associated with getting to sleep like thumbsucking, head rolling or hugging a special doll, stuffed animal, or piece of cloth. Older preschoolers who have learned to pace their activities may not need a nap or a prolonged period of rest; they may welcome a quiet time during the afternoon when they can lie down and listen to someone read aloud.

The children's rest periods give the staff time to relax in a separate place. Skillful scheduling provides sufficient rest for caregivers but assures that enough adults will be with the children to maintain order, take care of individual children's needs, and handle emergencies.

Scheduling adequate rest for children in the day care setting is important in teaching them to make a smooth transition from one activity to another. A quiet time between periods of strenuous play may make all the difference in the midpreschooler's ability to keep up. While scheduling for the child's performance in the day care program, planners must remember that the center's rest time will affect the child's conduct at home. Having a nap late in the day may make the child want to stay up beyond his usual bedtime at night; and lack of rest in the afternoon may cause him to be irritable during the short family time after dinner.

2.2.E Dressing

Dressing and undressing are activities that allow even the infant a chance to do for himself—to assist in putting an arm into a sleeve or lifting the buttocks for diaper changing. Toddlers and preschoolers can help in pulling on a jersey, zipping a snow suit, buttoning a shirt and tying shoes. All these acts require varying degrees of assistance. They should be accompanied by actions and words that instruct, encourage, and praise the child for his accomplishments. This is a good time for verbal communication.

2.2.F Activities Related to Personal Hygiene

Health promotion in any child care setting includes time for education and routines related to hand washing, use of the toilet, management of nasal secretions, and brushing of teeth. Self-care should be introduced according to the readiness of the child to participate both physically and cognitively.

2.2.G Activities for the School-Aged Child

Children who would be left to their own devices after school, commonly referred to as latch-key children, need a program of supervised activities designed specially for them. The school-aged child may need time after a day in the classroom for unregimented play, and space to run, climb, and jump. Children of this age are capable of sustained concentration and so welcome projects that may continue for an entire afternoon or for several days or weeks. They may do these projects alone or in groups.

Individual athletic activities or team sports may satisfy these children's desire to "work on something"; so may engaging in handcrafts or cooking, or producing a play. There are children who need or want supervision of homework or who prefer to write stories or read. In what they require, school-aged children tax the personal, physical, and financial resources of the day care center. Programs established primarily for preschool children may find it possible to satisfy only a fraction of the needs of the older child. Whether they can be run in separate facilities or not, programs for older children after school or during vacation time require additional skills and interests on the part of staff members beyond the personal qualities that all good caregivers share.

2.2.H Attitude Toward Sexuality

An unambivalent, factual attitude toward sexuality or the child's emerging sense of identity, shared by all their adult caregivers, creates a healthy atmosphere for children.[4] Developing a common approach to matters involving sexuality and identity is not always easy because the views of program administrators, staff members, parents, and community leaders do not always coincide.[5] Open discussion should be encouraged among the adults concerning childhood sexuality; and health providers and parents should feel comfortable asking questions of child care personnel regarding their attitude toward sexual identity and behavior prior to recommending or choosing a program for a child. Bias, restriction, or embarrassment regarding sex on the part of care providers may contribute to a child's feeling of anxiety related to sexuality.

Children learn about gender identification and sexual differences at the day care center as well as at home. Caregivers and parents should be reassured that interest in the genitals—their own and other children's—is normal for preschoolers. Adults should use common names and anatomically correct terms when referring to the children's genital organs, as they should when describing any part of the human body.[5]

Their developing awareness of gender is evident in the children's make-believe play. Caregivers can foster the preschooler's expression of feeling about the roles of male and female, and child and adult, by providing a housekeeping corner with clothing and homemaking props to facilitate the children's games. Play, which may include the assumption of roles such as mother, father, doctor, patient, and nurse, is expected and encouraged with active or passive participation of the adult caregiver—whichever appears to be needed in a particular situation. Dolls, both male and female, and other toys may be incorporated in the make-believe. Those toys associated with traditionally male and female activities frequently elicit the expression of entrenched adult bias about sex roles. Training by a health consultant can be helpful in learning techniques for clarifying staff and family attitudes toward sex roles and establishing a consistency for the purpose of reducing confusion for the child in care.

Masturbation is a normal expression of sexuality in both boys and girls from midinfancy onward, although there is a wide range of individual difference in its form and frequency. Decisions on management of this behavior ought to satisfy as far as possible both the parents and the day care staff members.[4] Most programs would prefer that masturbation be a private activity and children old enough to understand can be taught this. What may be considered excessive masturbation is a frequent concern of some child care providers. Health consultation to staff to describe the behavior of a particular child could be helpful. The health consultant may then assist staff in identifying activities that appear to increase the child's level of anxiety and withdrawal from a scheduled activity. Possible program adaptation to reduce stress, a change in group activity to increase enjoyment, and a suggestion to the parent for a health assessment may be advisable.

Physical contact between caregivers and the children is necessary to convey affection. Kissing, hugging, and cuddling infants and children is an expression of wholesome love that should be encouraged. Staff members may need assurance that such behavior will not be misinterpreted as sexual misconduct. In settings where this point is not made clear, the adults sometimes cease to embrace little boys when they move beyond the toddler stage. Certainly, there should be no improper physical handling of children, but caregivers should be advised to persist in their physical signs of affection for children of both sexes.[4]

2.3 Health Records

2.3.A The Child's Record

Day care health records should include information collected at registration as well as any new health and medical information that is received during the child's time in the program. (For sample Child Health Appraisal Forms, see Appendix II.1.) The frequency of health examinations is dependent upon the age of the infant or child and should follow the schedule established by the American Academy of Pediatrics unless there is a problem for which more frequent exams are indicated. A sample of Guidelines for Health Supervision is provided (Appendix V.2). State licensing requirements vary. Day care administrators should be familiar with the frequency of exams required in their state. For preschool children of migrant workers, day care may be the point of entry into the health care system. Migrant families should be encouraged to learn about health programs directed specifically to them.

The original record should always state why the child is in day care and the date of entry. It should include the child's date of birth, usual source of health care, and health payment resource. It should record the results of standard screening procedures (e.g., vision, hearing, Hbg./Hct., measurements, dentition, development) and the follow-up performed, in process, or needed. The record should document all immunizations and include a schedule for update, if necessary, and a health history from the parent and the primary health care provider. The results of a complete physical examination and an assessment of development should describe the child's state of physical health and level of function in the motor, cognitive, communicative, social, and emotional areas, with notations about unique characteristics that might require special adaptation of the day care program. The child's record should also include the composition of the family: the age and sex of siblings, the level of education of parents, their state of health, and their occupations. Any stresses in the home that may influence the child's behavior should be explained.

Children with known developmental disabilities should have an equally comprehensive record with recommendations for specific intervention, if needed, by a licensed qualified professional. Instructions should be written in language easily understood by the day care staff. Medical records should be considered to contain confidential data. The information is for the benefit of the child, family, and program. It is used for planning for the child, staffing needs, and determining eligibility. Records are particularly important for drop-in centers where there may be a need to trace contacts of a contagious disease. Records of children in night-time care should contain information regarding night-time sleep routines.

2.3.B Records of Medication and Diet

Every child care facility should have a written policy regarding the administration of medications. A sample Program Medication Administration Policy Form is provided in this manual (Appendix II.2). If a child requires medication at the day care center, that fact should be recorded. The record sheet should show the child's name, the name of the medication, the dose, the time when the medication is given, whether it requires refrigeration, and by whom it is administered. A sample Medication Checklist is provided in this manual (Appendix II.3). The record should include the reason for the medication, the name of the physician who prescribed it, and the parent's written consent to its use. A sample Medication Consent Form is provided in this manual (Appendix II.4). Medications not recommended by the child's physician should not be given in day care.

All children under 18 months of age should have documented specific diet instructions from the parent regarding formula, foods, and feeding schedule. Older children with special medical dietary needs or special diet supplements (e.g., Lofenalac) should have a descriptive statement in their record, written legibly (or typed), and signed by the person prescribing.

2.3.C Health Records for Staff, Substitutes, and Volunteers

There should be a health record for every adult who has contact with the children in the day care program or who is engaged in the preparation of food served to them. Besides a physical evaluation, preemployment examinations should provide an assessment of the individual's emotional fitness to be a caregiver. People whose mental state could pose a danger to children or whose health problems might be exacerbated by the requirements of the job should not be accepted as child care personnel. This rule applies to bus drivers, cooks, and secretaries, as well as to caregivers.

A sample Staff Health Appraisal Form is provided in this manual (Appendix II.5). Day care administrators using a form of their own design should be sure that it notes:

- Freedom from contagious disease.
- History of childhood infectious diseases such as rubella and chicken pox.
- Negative tuberculin test or, if positive, evidence of follow-up with a chest roentgenogram and evaluation for chemotherapy.
- Immunization status: types, initial dates, dates of boosters or reimmunizations (record of tetanus booster within ten years).
- Conditions that might cause frequent absence from the job.
- Conditions that might require emergency care.
- Limitations affecting performance of day care work (e.g., allergy to art materials, skin conditions affected by frequent hand washing, inability to stay outdoors).
- Medications and special diet requirements.
- Use of tobacco, alcohol, and drugs.
- Hearing and visual acuity.
- Evidence of mental and emotional fitness.
- Results of special tests for transporters including color and depth perception and size of the visual field.[6]

Health records of day care employees and volunteers should be updated by physical examinations every two years or as often as physicians advise on the basis of an individual's age and condition. In addition, a new examination is suggested when a person's health seems to be affecting job performance, when she or he returns to work after an injury, or when prolonged illness may necessitate at least a temporary modification of the caregiver's duties.

2.3.D Use of Health Records

Health care administrators should be aware that there are laws governing the confidentiality of health records, and use of records must be consistent with them. For example, The Family Rights and Privacy Act of 1974, a federal statute known informally as the Buckley Amendment, stipulates the permission of a parent or guardian before allowing access to the records of a child under the age of 18. (For a sample consent form, see Appendix II.6.) Because of the legal requirement of confidentiality and to prevent tampering with or damage to these important papers, health records should be kept in a safe place with restricted access.

Health records should be reviewed at the time of registration for the program by the health coordinator, and explanation of any irregularities should be sought from the program's health consultant or the child's primary health care provider. A decision as to whether the program can meet the child's needs should be made at that time.

Once a child has been admitted to the program, the information from the health profile helps the staff to plan a proper program. Knowing not only a healthy child's correct chronological age but also his developmental capacity prevents caregivers from expecting too much of a large child who looks older or from not allowing a small-sized one who looks younger to make decisions of which he is capable. It often helps to know that a young infant in the program was born prematurely, as these babies, although healthy, may not be as mature for their age as infants born at term. Having an assessment of a child's level of development allows the assignment of tasks that he or she can complete successfully: for instance, the less mature three-and-a-half-year-old who may not yet be able to cut on the line unassisted can be directed to tear the paper rather than be left to struggle with scissors.

With a complete health record in hand, caregivers can plan specifically for the child with chronic disease or special health needs. Documentation of diet and routine measurement of blood sugar level may be ordered for the child with diabetes; the medication schedule for an asthmatic child should be ascertained simply by reading his file. In health emergencies, the health care record serves as a valuable resource for the day care administrator who is communicating with an individual's family and primary health care provider.

2.4 Nutrition

2.4.A Feeding

Feeding is an essential health promotional day care activity. For the young infant, a caring familiar adult who is not rushed is important. A comfortable position for the infant and the person holding him or her, with opportunity to communicate both visually and verbally, contributes to the pleasure of the time together. As the child gains more voluntary control, his or her capacity to help in feeding should be encouraged and praised. Progress from holding a bottle, to eating with fingers, to holding a spoon, to drinking from a cup, to using utensils, is achievement that should be recognized. In the transition from mid- to late-infancy, some resistance to being fed comes with the striving for autonomy. Staff members should be reminded of the danger of propping a bottle for an infant because of the possibility of choking. Caregivers should also be reminded of the complications associated with the infant's drinking in a recumbent position and with falling asleep with a bottle of formula, milk, or juice in the mouth. The former may increase the incidence of otitis and the latter may result in the accelerated decay of teeth.

Most midinfancy children seated in adapted chairs will benefit from being part of a group at snack or meal time. Imitation is critical to development and contributes to social behavior at feeding time. The presence of an adult at the table who also eats the meal and encourages conversation about food, eating behaviors, and events of the day, adds to the desired pleasant atmosphere. This adult can assist the children in managing their food. She or he should be aware of the idiosyncrasies of individual children in food preference, portion size, and rate of eating, and be on the lookout for changes in eating habits that are indicators of poor health, either acute or chronic. Such changes would include irritability, refusal to eat, or reduction in usual appetite.

2.4.B Food Storage

Food purchased or accepted for use at a day care facility should be wholesome and unspoiled. Perishable foods should be kept clean and refrigerated. Cleanliness requires the use of new disposable or washed, sanitized containers, covered to keep out airborne particles. Food, including fluids like milk and juices, must never be returned from people's plates, cups, and drinking glasses to storage containers. Fresh milk and milk products should be pasteurized and refrigerated at a temperature between 37° and 45°F. To check the maintenance of proper temperature in a refrigerator without a built-in thermometer, a thermometer can be placed in a cup of water in the refrigerator 12 inches from the door.

Drinking water need not be refrigerated. It can be stored in or near the rooms occupied by the children. It should be held in closed containers to prevent contamination and served in clean cups like other fluids. Reusable cups, like reusable dishes, should be washed and sanitized after each use.

2.4.C Management of Meals

Age-appropriate types of foods must be available. Food should be presented at meals, snack, and special times, never as a reward or punishment. Children should be encouraged but not forced to eat. Ethnic preferences and familiarity affect a child's adaptability to the day care menu. Good management of meals can minimize resistance to eating a variety of foods: portions that are not too large or small, safe chairs and tables of the right size, and the presence of caregivers who talk and help, all contribute to the children's willingness to eat the food that is served. If possible, enough food for "seconds" should be allowed, and meal times should be unhurried. A rotating menu prepared by a dietician may offer nutritious foods in sufficient variety to encourage good eating habits and avoid the boredom of repetition.[7]

Babies just beginning to feed themselves require close supervision. To prevent choking they should be given one bite at a time of foods of proper size, shape, and consistency. "Squirreling" of several pieces of food increases the likelihood of choking. Foods such as peanuts may pass through the larynx and occlude the lower airway. Chunks of hot dogs and grapes, for example, may completely occlude the upper airway. Presence of molars is a good indication of a healthy child's ability to chew hard foods such as raw carrots and many candies that are likely to cause choking.[8] If toddlers walk around while eating or drinking from a bottle, choking will occur more easily. A fall with the bottle in the toddler's mouth can cause dental injury.

The management of meals for infants and children with feeding problems takes special care. Special equipment, like body support mechanisms and tube-feeders, and special techniques for positioning may be required to deliver food to infants and children with specific feeding problems. The presence of the child with such a problem at the day care facility requires staff members willing and able to cope with the situation. The administrator must be able to spare these caregivers for considerable periods of time and to provide instruction for them by parents, physicians, community nurses, or other developmental specialists (e.g., occupational therapists or physical therapists).

Infants still entirely dependent on milk or formula may not be amenable to a strict feeding schedule. Some can be fed at specific times but others may sleep for five hours or more and then want more frequent feedings. It is important to allow for flexibility in the routine because babies vary in their desire to be fed. Caregivers and parents should keep each other aware of a child's change in feeding pattern and adapt to it.

Milk or formula may be provided by the day care center or the parent, but formula prepared at home and carried to the center should be discouraged. If disposable nursers are not used, the milk or formula should be poured into clean bottles supplied by the parent or bottles sanitized in the dishwasher at the care facility. Bottles should be labeled with the child's name. The feeding process should not be rushed; feeding should be considered complete when the infant finishes steady sucking. Milk left in the bottle should be discarded. If parents insist on bringing formula from home, safe transport and feeding is best achieved when concentrated liquid or powdered formula is provided. It should be suggested that measuring and mixing can then be done at the day care site just prior to feeding.

If a mother decides to continue breastfeeding, caregivers should be supportive and try to adapt to the parent's schedule. The mother may come to the day care center once or several times during the day or she may leave breast milk in bottles to be stored in the refrigerator until needed. Caregivers must be sure that a mother supplying her breast milk in a bottle has collected, stored, and transported it using sanitary techniques. (For recommendations for collecting and storing breast milk, see Appendix II.7.)

2.4.D Diet

Meals and snacks should be designed to supply children's dietary requirements for good health.[7,9] Unless a dietician is on the staff, it would be advisable to consult a qualified nutritionist or a food service specialist in planning the content of meals. (For a general guide to content and size of portions, see Appendix II.8.) Types of food appropriate for each age group should be selected; but whatever the menu, each meal for toddlers and preschool children should contain at least one item from each of the following food groups:

• Dairy products: milk, cheese, cream, yogurt
• Protein: meat, poultry, fish, eggs, cheese, peanut butter, peas, dried beans, nuts
• Fruits and vegetables: all types
• Grains: whole grains and enriched grain products such as bread, cereals, crackers, pasta, rice

Children with food allergies or other conditions requiring a special diet must be served in accordance with the regimen described over the signature of the physician on the order in the child's health record. Vitamin supplements also must be provided as prescribed by written order of the physician. Consultation with parents and the health care provider is advisable before introducing new foods into the diet of an infant for whom no instructions are on file. No nutritional advantage results from the introduction of supplemental foods prior to four to six months of age. The specific time depends on the infant's ability to sit with support and with good control of head and neck. The child will then be able to open his or her mouth, lean forward, and turn his or her head away.[10]

The quantity of food provided should satisfy but not exceed daily requirements. The distribution of food should be guided by a time schedule. If a child is in day care for

- 3 to 4 hours (either in midmorning or the afternoon): he/she should be given a snack timed no closer than two hours before the next scheduled meal.
- 5 to 8 hours: he/she should receive one third to one half of the total daily food requirement given in one or more servings.
- 9 hours or more: he/she should receive at least two thirds of the total daily requirement in the form of two meals and two snacks.[9]

2.5 Control of Behavior

To foster social development, a day care program should have a clearly defined code of behavior and a disciplinary policy to support it. Good behavior should be elicited in a positive and kind way—never by inflexible, punitive measures that instill fear. Because corporal punishment can inflict physical and psychological harm, it must not be condoned in any child care setting.

Behavioral goals and disciplinary methods established for the program should be explained to new caregivers and to parents because not everyone shares the same opinion about what is "right." It is important for staff members to be consistent in their approach, and the best results are achieved with family cooperation.

Children have to be given understandable guidelines for their behavior if they are to develop internal control of their actions. The aim is to develop personal standards and self-discipline, not to enforce a set of institutional rules. Verbal explanations are important, particularly during the second and third years when the child's understanding of language enables him or her to understand the verbal explanation. They are time consuming but they enable a child to generalize from a specific incident and thus to learn for the future from current experience. Caregivers must not focus only on infractions; they should be quick to recognize good behavior and to reward it with praise.

Day care administrators and caregivers can facilitate good behavior by creating an environment responsive to the children's needs. A good "fit" between the temperament of the caregiver and the child always helps. Allowing adequate rest and timing meals and snacks properly prevents children from becoming overtired and hungry and thus more likely to misbehave. Placing children in competition for toys or the attention of too small a number of caregivers also encourages antisocial actions. The cause of a child's persistent poor behavior should be explored. If staff cannot correct the problem with changes in the child care environment, consultation with an outside professional with parental permission should be recommended. Maintaining a setting in which good behavior is attained without visible "punishment" contributes significantly to decreasing later psychological and behavioral disorders. Children cared for inadequately at home, a group that contributes disproportionately to the 40% of school children with psychobehavioral disorders, can particularly benefit from such a day care setting.

2.6 Helping the Parent in the Use of Day Care

It is not the intent of this manual to advocate day care over in-home parent care when home care is nurturing and supportive to the needs of the growing child. Day care is generally thought of as a regularly scheduled acceptable supplement to the care provided to a child by parents who are employed. Day care may also supplement the care provided by parents who for a variety of other reasons are not available to their children for many hours of the day. The parents may be teenagers who wish to continue education or vocational training. A parent may be physically or mentally ill and require regular child care services. A parent may have many scheduled appointments with a variety of services on a regular basis. A parent may not be able to provide nurturing care because of great personal stress. Or a parent may not have the capacity to provide prolonged continuing care without outside help.

Pediatricians should help parents in their practice to understand that regardless of the reason for their use of a child care facility, they should be involved in all decisions affecting their child while he or she is there. Daily contacts are easier in some settings than others. Staff in large centers with long hours have shifts of personnel so that the person greeting the child in the morning may not be on duty in the afternoon. It is generally easier to have daily contact with the primary caregiver in a family day care home. Parents of children who are transported to the child care facility by nonfamily members need to make other arrangements for communication. Periodic conferences can be scheduled. Some child care providers make home visits. Notes can be exchanged. Formal group meetings of parents and staff should be encouraged for discussing individual children and to offer knowledge of such topics as stages of child development and common childhood behaviors and their management, both at home and in the child care setting. Such parent support by day care staff may be an entry point for some families to other needed social and health services. The importance of the parent's relationship with the child should always be respected.

Guidelines for judging day care settings have been established (see Appendix II.9). The best measure of the success of a particular program is consistent, sequential development of each child who participates in the daily activities with enjoyment. Regression in development or reduction in rate of physical, social, or psychological development should be assessed immediately and thoroughly by the family, the center staff, and if persistent, the child's physician.

Pediatricians should be active not only in educating their patients' families about the characteristics of a program of good quality, but also in advocating an adequate number and variety of programs within their communities which meet such criteria. They should help parents to look for the right program for their child.[11] They should also refer parents to resource and referral centers that are developing in communities around the country to offer information, encourage the development of needed services, and advocate services of good quality.

2.7. Conclusion

No single recommendation made in this chapter is less important than the others for the maintenance of the health and well-being of the child in day care. Good day care programs already embody many of them in some form; physicians and other health care providers can help to improve care programs in their communities by suggesting ways to execute them more effectively. Evidence of success lies in the progress of the children's physical, social, and psychological development. Good results are worth working for.

References

1. Haggerty RJ, Roghmann KJ, Pless IB: *Child Health and the Community.* New York, Interscience Series, John Wiley & Sons, Inc, 1975, pp 94-95
2. Prescott E, David TG: The effects of the physical environment on day care. Concept paper in the review of the appropriateness of the federal interagency day care requirements. Washington, DC Office of the Assistant Secretary for Planning and Evaluation, Department of Health, Education, and Welfare, July 1976 (unpublished)
3. Provence S: *Guide for the Care of Infants in Groups.* New York, Child Welfare League of America, 1967
4. Constantine LL, Martinson FM: *Children and Sex. New Findings, New Perspectives.* Boston, Little, Brown and Company, 1981
5. Gordon S, Gordon J: *Raising a Child Conservatively in a Sexually Permissive World,* New York, Simon and Schuster, 1983, Chapters 4 and 6
6. Aronson SS: Health Update, Why is Adult Health An Issue in Day Care? *Child Care Information Exchange,* March 1984

7. Hille HM: *Food for Groups of Young Children Cared for during the Day.* DHEW Publication No. 386. Washington, DC: US Government Printing Office, 1960

8. *Foods and Choking in Children* (a report to the Food and Drug Administration on a conference held in Elkridge, MD, August 4-5, 1983). Evanston, IL, American Academy of Pediatrics, December 1983

9. *Handbook for Local Head Start Nutrition Specialists.* DHHS Publication No. (OHDS) 84-31189. Washington, DC: US Government Printing Office, 1983

10. Committee on Nutrition: *Pediatric Nutrition Handbook.* ed 2. Elk Grove Village, IL, American Academy of Pediatrics, 1985, pp 28-31

11. Dittmann L: *Children in Day Care with Focus on Health.* Washington, DC: US Government Printing Office, DHEW Publication No. 444, 1967

Chapter 3

DAY CARE FOR THE CHILD WITH SPECIAL NEEDS

3.1 Introduction

Children who have developmental disabilities or a chronic illness need day care as much, if not more, than their nondisabled peers. Although day care programs for these children are available in some areas, most of these infants and children still do not have access to the day care they would have if they were normal. Day care and other community services which facilitate the development of such children and enable their families to function better should be advocated and assisted by pediatricians and physicians in family practice.

3.2 The Improving Prognosis for Children with Developmental Disabilities

The extent to which disabled children have been served in the community has grown since the implementation in 1978 of Public Law 94-142, the Education for All Handicapped Children Act. Since early and appropriate intervention has been made available, the prognosis has improved for the eventual independence or semi-independence of these children. Many infants who score poorly on early neurodevelopmental tests or are designated "at risk" because of perinatal complications now recover or improve. Some eventually develop to a level that allows learning and behavior within normal limits. With the development of programs for early detection and intervention in many communities over the past two decades, some children with disorders such as Down Syndrome, which formerly led to institutionalization, now develop the adaptive, cognitive, and social skills necessary to succeed in community employment as adults, while living in semi-independent or independent settings.[1]

This kind of improvement does not occur accidentally. Children do not just "outgrow" their handicaps without intervention. They need training and experience at home, at school, and in other settings where they can develop required skills and learn to handle responsibilities. Their families require guidance and support.

The prognosis of many children with syndromes known to be associated with developmental disabilities can no longer be determined by the physician in a single evaluation. A more comprehensive interdisciplinary assessment is recommended to plan an effective intervention program. The child needs periodic reevaluation to determine the extent to which the program is succeeding. Modifications may be necessary as a child's progress is monitored because much is yet unknown about the factors that cause or affect certain disabilities. For instance, it has been commonly assumed that anoxia during birth is responsible for reduced intellectual function observed later in development; yet recent studies of children with and without signs of perinatal anoxia have shown that differences in measured intellectual levels seem to relate more to the socio-economic status of the subjects than the presence or absence of anoxia.[2] It is uncertain whether these results are related to a lack of access to adequate day care and infant stimulation programs for infants of families at lower socio-economic levels.

3.3 Integrating Disabled with Nondisabled Children

When day care is deemed advisable for a disabled child, health advisors and family should seek a program that follows the basic guidelines for day care service, described elsewhere in this manual. Whether disabled children are integrated with nondisabled children or cared for separately, special programming and equipment may be required. Although special arrangements may necessitate extra effort or financial outlay, there is good reason for admitting children with disabilities to programs designed for nondisabled children.[3]

When it can be achieved, the integration of young disabled and nondisabled children has advantages for both groups. This is not a new concept. Several years after the inception of Head Start in 1965, programs were mandated to include a minimum of 10% of the handicapped children in the populations served. Local programs still vary, however, in the severity of the handicapping conditions with which they can cope; care providers are faced with children whose problems range from mild speech disorders to a multitude of severe disabilities. Certain outstanding day care centers and Early Childhood Education programs for developmentally disabled children have served as models of integrated facilities. The Waisman Center in Madison, Wisconsin has such a demonstration program. Another was developed by an affiliate of the Rose F. Kennedy Center in the Bronx, New York. A third was begun in 1980 as a Saturday program by faculty and special education students of York University in Toronto, Canada. The Saturday program grew into a summer program and eventually became the Thousand Cranes School, a school in which handicapped and nonhandicapped children are educated together, with both individualized and group work for each child. All children benefit from their experience in an integrated center. Developmentally disabled children benefit from having relationships with peers in the mainstream, and normal children develop sensitivity, respect, and friendship for individuals who, aside from their physical problems, are quite like them. In short, integration of disabled and nondisabled children works well; it requires a very skillful child care staff to assure that the needs of each child in the heterogeneous group are met.[4]

3.4 The Role of the Pediatrician in Day Care for Children with Disabilities

3.4.A Referral

Pediatricians should be sensitive to the needs of children and families in their practices and know when to recommend day care. The indications for day care for children with disabilities are similar to those for any children—the need for care, supervision, structure, stimulation, training, and peer interaction, to supplement that provided by the parents. Both parents or the single parent may work, a parent may be ill and unable to care for the child, or she or he may merely need to participate in some non-child-care activities which will permit both parent and child to return home better able to live, work, and play together. One or both parents of a disabled child may be depressed and temporarily lack the emotional and physical energy to care for the child on a 24-hour basis. (Parents of normal children rarely must care intensively for their children as many hours a day as parents of children who are disabled.) Parents of children with disabilities may need day care more than others and are less likely to find it.

3.4.B Advocacy

The pediatrician may not find satisfactory day care for disabled patients available at the time it is needed. If the child with disabilities does not seem to fit into any particular group, the pediatrician may have to support the parents in their efforts to secure it. Sometimes such support involves testifying at a public hearing or before a state legislature for the necessity of providing funds or facilities. More often, the physician can work directly with the administrators of existing programs, suggesting modifications to accommodate the child. Both parents and day care personnel may want advice—whether to place a mentally retarded child with children of his mental or chronological age, for instance, or how to manage a child with a seizure or other acute medical problem. Advocacy may take the form of education, such as explaining a child's disabling condition or convincing a care provider that a child can be served with age mates despite his being behind in the development of self-help skills.

Advocating the best day care for a disabled child should involve visiting a facility to judge firsthand whether it can meet the current developmental needs of a particular child or visiting more than one center to determine which setting would be the best one for him. Familiarizing himself or herself with day care programs in the community will enable the physician to suggest alternative care settings as the needs of the patient and his family change. Planning has to be long-range because a child with disabilities may require day or after-school care longer than nondisabled peers.

3.4.C Program Consultation and Support

A day care program serving one or more children with disabilities may require more support by the pediatrician than other day care settings. The pediatrician may be asked to participate on a board or advisory committee and so have an opportunity to advocate on the supervisory level. The effectiveness of such a board or committee will be increased as its members gain a better understanding of the day care program and the concerns of its administrators and staff as well as the needs of the disabled children and their families. Physicians can contribute in staff development sessions on the early detection and management of disabling conditions in the day care setting, or make periodic health and safety visits in order to identify potential problems that have been overlooked. Physicians should recommend the institution or modification of policies and procedures to facilitate the health and safety of all children. When external (or internal) regulations become barriers to service rather than supports, the pediatrician may be of assistance in obtaining the modifications or exceptions necessary to insure excellent day care for children with and without disabilities.

3.5 Pediatric Care and Support of Children with Disabilities and Their Families

Pediatric care for children with disabilities or chronic health problems must be comprehensive and continuing. An assessment may require sequential examinations to establish a diagnosis and to determine both medical and developmental needs. The care also must include a case management component and the physician must be an active participant in it. That is, the pediatrician, in addition to providing guidance in health promotion and the treatment of illnesses as they occur, should offer a more comprehensive annual (or, if necessary, even a more frequent) review and conference with child, parents, and child care staff. Topics considered should include the child's present status, recent changes and prognosis regarding physical and emotional health, disabling condition(s), growth, development, and concerns of parents and child care staff regarding behavior in various settings and situations. Consultations held since the last conference, including those with other professionals who also care for the child, should be noted, and all results and recommendations should be reviewed in affirming or revising the child's program.

In a conference, parents should be encouraged to set forth their current plans, hopes, and goals for their child. The physician should be especially supportive as parents express themselves because they frequently have difficulty in clarifying what they expect or in discussing and accepting limitations that affect what they want for their child and their family. When they lack sufficient information to make plans or to know what they can hope for realistically, the pediatrician should recommend ways for them to obtain more objective data before the next conference. There should also be thorough coverage of old and new problems with regard to the extent to which they are likely to impede the child's physical, emotional, and cognitive development. An assessment ought to be made, also, of the child's interactions with family members, day care staff, teachers, and peers. Throughout the discussion, care should be taken to help parents and caregivers avoid erroneously attributing a treatable behavior problem or illness to the handicapping condition. The physician should identify these factors and prescribe aggressive treatment to eliminate or minimize the episodic, recurrent or persistent medical illness or behavior dysfunction that is interfering with the child's growth and development.

It should also be remembered that infants and very young children go through a period when they form attachments to their caregivers and learn to trust others to provide for their needs. Limitation of the total number of primary caregivers has been shown to facilitate this process. Young handicapped children go through the same process which may be prolonged as a result of underlying psychological and cognitive delays. Provision of services to such children often involves the participation of many people with special skills. As a result, there is an increase in the number of adults caring for a given child. Special effort should be made to limit the number of staff members who act as caregivers in such situations. One way to keep the number low is to have specialists work with a few primary caregivers (perhaps even a single individual) who deal directly with the child.

Many schools and programs for children with disabilities require interdisciplinary annual reviews. Collaboration among parents, physicians, teachers, consultants, and day care staff facilitates the rehabilitation of handicapped children in the most normal and least restrictive environment possible. The pediatrician is in a unique position in these conferences to be an informed advocate for the child with disabilities in day care, assuring him or her an opportunity for early development of the skills and relationships that will be crucial throughout life.

3.6 Provision for Children with Specific Disabilities

In addition to general procedures to be followed for disabled children in day care, there are special adaptations associated with specific kinds of handicapping conditions.

3.6.A The Child with Sensory Impairment

Caregivers entrusted with a child whose sight or hearing is impaired need, besides the child's general health records, special instruction from a professional concerning the implications of the sensory loss. Whether it is the child's primary care physician or an ophthalmologist, optometrist, otologist, or audiologist, there must be someone who explains what the child perceives, the problems he will encounter in the day care setting, and the kind of assistance he should and should not have. The use or operation of the child's sensory aids should be explained. It should be emphasized that the child has to be protected from harm, but, at the same time, encouraged to function as independently as possible.

Day care administrators should be given some direction in finding specialists who can assess sensory function and make suggestions for adaptations of existing facilities that will be of help to children with visual or auditory impairments. Such specialists may be available through public service programs at the state or local level in departments of public health or special education.

3.6.B The Child with Neuromotor or Skeletal Abnormalities

Disabilities of this kind, involving obligatory reflexes, muscle paralysis, weakness, spasticity, missing limbs, or congenital malformations, most commonly produce problems of mobility and posture, requiring special equipment and special care. The physical character of the day care center must allow use of the child's supportive devices and staff members must be trained to manipulate them. Staff persons will need to communicate regularly with the providers of rehabilitative services to the specific child to learn feeding and holding techniques, exercises, and other special procedures in order to maintain and promote health. Adaptations may be necessary in the care center's program to gear cognitive, communicative, and social activities to the child's capacity.

3.6.C The Child with Chronic Illness

Chronic illness is a broad category that includes, as disorders commonly seen in children, asthma, severe allergies, diabetes, seizures, heart disease, and sickle cell anemia. Without describing at length the needs of children with each of these conditions, it is possible to recommend basic rules that apply in every case.

The physician should alert the parents and the child's caregivers to symptoms of the disease, emphasizing those that require immediate attention when they appear. Those that the caregiver can manage should be distinguished from those that necessitate the services of a physician. Instructions for contacting the appropriate health professional in emergencies, or simply for asking questions about management, should be left in writing. Also in writing in the child's file there should be directions for medications or special diets to be followed during the day care period. In counseling caregivers in or out of the home, the physician should try to ease anxiety by explaining how to cope with routine problems and stressing his or her availability.

The child with a chronic illness may require restrictions in his program. For example, a child with an uncorrected heart problem, not having the endurance of his peers, may need additional rest, more frequent small meals, or shorter active play periods. For the child's psychological health, however, it is important that he feel as much as possible like a normal member of his group. For that reason, the physician and the child's parents should encourage child care personnel not to restrict a child in ways other than those that have been specifically prescribed.

References

1. Bricker DD: *Intervention with At Risk and Handicapped Infants*, Baltimore, MD, University Park Press, 1982
2. Sameroff AJ, Chandler MJ: Reproductive risk and the continuum of caretaking casualty. FD Horowitz (ed): *Review of Child Development Research*. Vol. 4. University of Chicago Press, 1975, pp 187-244
3. Packer R: Integrated day care: service delivery options that really work!—Paper presented at meeting of Region V American Association of Mental Deficiency, Alexandria, LA, October 1985 (unpublished)
4. Kieran SS, Connor FP, Von Hippel CS, Jones SH: *Mainstreaming Preschoolers: Children with Orthopedic Handicaps*, A guide for teachers, parents, and others who work with orthopedically handicapped preschoolers. DHHS Publication No. (OHDS) 81-31114, Reprinted. Washington, DC, US Government Printing Office, 1981

Chapter 4

DAY CARE AND CHILD ABUSE

4.1 Introduction

Child abuse is known to occur in any setting where children may be. The only essential conditions for child abuse are the presence of the vulnerable child, the presence of the person prone to abuse, and one of a variety of immediate situational circumstances. All children are vulnerable to abuse; some more than others. Many persons are prone to abuse children because they were themselves abused as children. The most important environmental circumstance which favors abuse is isolation.

The scope of the problem has always been difficult to assess. Much depends upon definitions plus a willingness to perceive the problem, and many rather civilized countries deny its existence.[1] There have been some dramatic recent changes in the level of concern, due in part to increases in the reporting of sexual abuse.[2] Physical abuse may be showing a real increase in incidence in the 1980s. In 1979 R.S. and C.H. Kempe could write that the number of hospitalized children who died of child abuse in Denver had dropped from about 20 to just one case in a year.[3] Similarly, in San Diego no deaths at all were attributed to abuse at the Children's Hospital in 1979. In 1985, however, the number of deaths returned to the higher levels experienced 20 years earlier.

Child abuse and neglect in all its forms is still a less frequent cause of death and major injury than accidents, especially automobile accidents, but there is nothing that does more lasting harm to more infants and children. Much of the harm takes the form of very long-term impairment of functioning related to emotional and cognitive developmental disturbances, rather than obvious physical disability.[4]

Because the harm caused by child abuse is serious and undeniable, it is necessary to design preventive measures even though the occurrence of child abuse has not yet been conclusively delineated and quantified. It is known that abuse may take place in children's own homes, in institutions, in foster homes, in schools, in the offices of physicians, psychologists, and dentists who care for children, and in all sorts of child care settings. An unclear picture of the incidence of child abuse has emerged because of erratic reporting, inadequate verification, and, in some cases, sensational publicity. Even without accurate data, however, there are still steps that can be taken through day care programs to reduce child abuse: day care personnel can eliminate the possibility of abuse on their own premises, recognize and rescue children who are suffering it elsewhere, and provide a haven for children who are likely to be abused at home.

4.2 The Occurrence of Abuse in Day Care

Understanding of how abuse occurs in day care settings is far from complete and is largely based upon accounts of individual cases and testimony usually distorted by the needs of the adult participants to protect themselves. The ages of the child victims often preclude obtaining exact and precise descriptions of events. The problem of defensive distortion can sometimes be solved by substituting treatment for punishment for certain sorts of offenders, but this solution applies more readily to intrafamilial abusers than to abusers of children in day care. The problem of obtaining good histories from very young, preverbal children has been partially overcome by the increasing use of play techniques in interviewing them and by increasing knowledge and skill applied to the physical examination.

Child abuse does not lend itself to structured, objective studies. When it is discovered, it must be terminated; it cannot be observed or analyzed as it occurs "naturally." Therefore, knowledge of abuse is built up through multiple case histories. Enough of these have accumulated from the day care setting to allow some cautious generalization. The differences between physical abuse and sexual abuse are sufficiently great (despite some overlap) to require separate characterization of the two types.

4.2.A Physical Abuse

Physical abuse occurs in day care under conditions quite similar to those under which it occurs in natural homes. A person predisposed to abuse children, often because of an abusive experience in childhood, commits the abusive acts during a time of stress, usually while other adults are not at hand. The abuse presents itself as signs of injury with a discrepant history.

Poorly staffed day care centers and family day care homes, where isolated caregivers are burdened with more children than they can manage, are more likely to have abuse occur than at adequately staffed facilities where stressful situations can be coped with more readily and other adults are present to observe the inappropriate behavior.

Physical abuse of children under an adult's care is not always unintentional or the result of sudden anger. Deliberate physical abuse has been reported more frequently in the last few years (although it has doubtless been going on for a long time). Some individuals have a strong belief in the necessity of corporal punishment as a component of child management. They see its limitation in a group setting as a restriction of that right. A group of such persons may organize a child care system and employ harsh physical punishment. If the group is religiously affiliated, this may not be prohibited in states where church-sponsored child care programs have a religious exemption from state standards.[5]

4.2.B Sexual Abuse

Unlike physical abuse, which usually occurs in an explosive, unplanned fashion, sexual abuse very frequently is carefully planned for days, weeks, or months before the actual acts. Persons of either sex who are sexually attracted to children often seek employment or volunteer in occupations that bring them into close contact with children. Once so employed, they work to gain the confidence of children, parents, and other staff members and very frequently gain that confidence. Only then do they begin, privately and secretly, to commit sexual acts with the children entrusted to them.

Individual employees or volunteers at day care centers may sexually abuse children, but because opportunities for privacy at most centers are difficult to secure, help or collusion from another employee may be necessary.

4.3 Recognition of Abuse Occurring in Day Care

4.3.A Physical Abuse

Physical abuse occurring in day care presents itself in the same way as it does in other settings (see Appendix IV.1). Usually, some person other than the abuser recognizes signs of injuries that are either clearly nonaccidental or are unlikely to have occurred in the manner or at a time stated by the caregiver. When the injuries are not serious, the parent may see them first after undressing a child for a bath at the end of a day during which the child was in care. When the injuries are serious, the provider usually calls for medical assistance but gives an inaccurate history of the events causing the injury. In either case, the problem that results is often a complex medicolegal one that requires careful and skilled investigation by law enforcement and/or protective services persons assisted by medical evidentiary examination. Usually, a licensing agency also needs to be involved. Many cases remain unresolved because of medical inability to fix a time of injury with sufficient precision to distinguish objectively between an injury produced at home and in a day care setting.

A rather rare but harrowing occurrence is that of more than one instance of sudden unexpected infant death occurring in the same day care setting in a relatively short space of time, perhaps less than one year. Since there is no medical method to distinguish between sudden infant death syndrome (SIDS) and deliberate suffocation, the investigators are left with epidemiological inferences and statistical probabilities. Under these conditions, it is difficult to make firm recommendations; however, a conservative position would be that any provider who has an occurrence of SIDS in his or her care should be under close surveillance by the licensing agency. If additional cases occur, a calculation of the likelihood that they are true SIDS is quite simple, based upon the number of infants cared for, the passage of time and the known incidence of SIDS. This may be the only objective basis for a decision about continuing licensure since surveillance for other possibly abusive events is unlikely to be helpful.

4.3.B Sexual Abuse

Sexual abuse occurring in day care may go unrecognized for long periods of time because of the skill of the perpetrators in avoiding discovery and in making the victims keep the secret. When the victims are under four years of age, they may give an indication of the existence of the abuse by showing age-inappropriate sexual behavior, regressive or disturbed behavior, or problems associated with the genital area or the anus, including venereal diseases (gonorrhea, herpes, venereal warts, or vaginal discharge caused by several different organisms), abnormalities of the labial skin, bleeding from the vaginal or anal area, or fecal soiling in children previously free of fecal accidents. When the victims are able to tell their story in words, they may do so at all sorts of unexpected times; but they may only do so once if they are not taken seriously. Almost invariably, they are under some form of coercion by the perpetrator to keep the secret. Older children who are being abused but who are afraid to tell may demonstrate a variety of altered behaviors related to almost intolerable stress.[6] Any child whose previously healthy behavior patterns change without explanation should be considered to be a possible victim of sexual abuse and a sensitive inquiry should be made into the possibility. Children who begin to express serious distress about being left in day care should have their concerns considered thoughtfully. If such behavior develops anew in a child who has previously tolerated separation well, it should be taken very seriously.

When a child is brought to attention because of one of the behavioral changes that may indicate sexual abuse or with genital or anal signs, the physician or counselor usually has no immediate way of knowing whether to be concerned about the home, the day care source, or still another setting. For this reason it is very unwise (although often irresistible) to attempt to resolve the problem without assistance from a protective or law enforcement agency. This principle becomes even more important when a child begins, in the day care setting, to demonstrate behaviors indicative of abuse. If the care facility employs a number of workers, the one making the observation may have no way of telling whether or not another employee is molesting the child or if the abuse is occurring at home. Looking into a situation of this kind requires great skill and a level of objectivity that usually cannot be provided within the organization where the problem exists.

4.4 Prevention of Child Abuse in Day Care

When an instance of abuse in day care is reported, there is a tendency to advocate an increase in the inspection capabilities of the licensing agencies. This is desirable, but perhaps not obtainable everywhere. Indeed, some states do not require family day care providers to be licensed and do not regulate them in any way.[5] While professional organizations should continue to work for improved licensing and inspection, they should also recognize that the most important preventive methods that can be applied to abuse in day care are still those of selection of the care facility and monitoring by parents and observation of caregivers' performance by their peers.

4.4.A Advice to Parents

There are many brochures and booklets that tell parents how to select a source of child care. (A very complete one has been published by the U.S. Department of Health and Human Services. See Appendix II.9, checklist #1.) Most of them emphasize a careful evaluation of the provider prior to acceptance, using inspection, interview, references, and recommendations. Many fail to mention what may be the most important safeguard that the parent has: the unscheduled visit. Parents should have an advance agreement with the provider that they may visit at any time, and they should do so as long as the child is in care. The visits need not be frequent and they certainly can be brief. The parent has an obligation not to be disruptive, but he or she should see the child and assess the setting and what is going on in it each time. Another useful technique is to get acquainted with other parents who use the same provider and occasionally share experiences in semisocial meetings or over the phone.

By these methods, as well as the standard ones described in brochures, parents can be satisfied that they have done about all they can do to prevent the abuse of their children in day care. Some abuse will still occur, and parents, providers, and helping professionals all share a responsibility to continue to work for the total elimination of it.

4.4.B Advice to Providers

Providers need to gain some understanding of the thought processes and beliefs of those caregivers who are likely to abuse children. In the case of physical abuse, it is likely that the person who commits it, in most cases, does not know in advance that he or she is going to do so. What abusers may know is that they were themselves abused in childhood. They may also know that some aspects of looking after infants or children of certain ages cause them to feel inadequate or to experience other sorts of distress. For such people the profession of child care is an unwise choice. For a person already "trapped" in such a choice, a first precaution is to try never to be alone with children when feeling bad; the next thing is to try to find other work. Resolving the problems caused by having been abused as a child is difficult and time consuming and best done when away from the pressures of child care. Whereas these recommendations may seem harsh, they are much less so than the consequences of being proven to have physically abused an infant.

Center operators must be conscious of the existence of pedophilia and the techniques employed by pedophiles to gain private access to children, as well as of the behaviors of children who are being sexually abused. As yet, there is no reliable method for screening potential employees for this problem; but it is perfectly legal to ask about it in a preemployment interview in many states, and this practice might have some value. Criminal record checks and fingerprinting for providers are being required in some states,[7] but whether or not these rather expensive measures are effective is still unknown.

Policies and practices which eliminate private access of adults to children in care are very wise. All employees should know that they may be visited at any time by the director or by a parent. Center staff should all be instructed about child sexual abuse.

Family day care providers who employ assistants or who allow access to children by their relatives or friends must use the same care in selecting such persons as operators of larger facilities do in hiring.

Conscientious, nonabusive providers should not be fearful of being accused of sexual abuse because of physical contact with children that is normal and necessary in providing care. Neither should they let themselves be inhibited from holding, hugging, and personal contact with infants and young children who need it. It is quite simple to tell the difference between the affectionate holding of children and sexual abuse. The latter, when young children are victims, almost always involves at least touching of the child's genitals or the anal area while the perpetrator seeks sexual arousal or gratification. (Sexual involvement with adolescent children may be quite different, but this is unlikely to arise in the day care setting.) Because most providers of day care are conscientious and truly concerned with children's welfare, it is likely that day care settings will come to be recognized as places in which knowledge about sexual abuse is applied to prevent it.

4.5 Reporting

The reporting requirement for persons who are professionally involved with children, in most states, is based upon the suspicion of abuse. In most states persons who work with children are required to report abuse and are referred to as "mandated reporters." Mandated reporters are not required to prove their allegations; however, there are many reasons why reports should be carefully made. Considerable harm may come to the person who is the subject of the report if the report is incorrect; the victims also may be harmed by the investigative process, and the agencies responsible for investigating reports are often overwhelmed by the volume of work presented to them, with the result that cases may not be carefully explored.

Many states now have reporting laws that require that the information be given only to law enforcement or child protective agencies. In such states, reporters of abuse occurring in day care may be legally prevented from notifying the families using the facility in which the abuse occurred.

Providers of care to families are typically reluctant to report child abuse in the families they serve. Day care providers are no exception to this general rule. In San Diego County (pop. 2,000,000) in 1983, of 26,000 reports of child abuse and neglect, 86, or less than 1% were made by day care providers of all kinds. Given the fact that 15% to 20% of children are receiving some form of day care, there are probably cases of abuse being overlooked in the day care setting just as there are in schools and doctors' offices. Day care providers could be more helpful in detecting abuse if they were trained to recognize and report instances that occur.

Persons reporting for the first time are wise to seek advice from others with more experience. Familiarity with state laws and local arrangements for the reporting of child abuse is obligatory for all persons who work with children.

4.6 Investigation

A detailed description of how investigations of abuse should be carried out is beyond the scope of this chapter; however, a few observations are in order. Investigations of cases of possible physical abuse have been made in large numbers for many years and many communities have systems of interacting medical and protective agencies that function fairly well. The system for investigating sexual abuse is much more primitive, and there are still wide variations between the systems in different places. Methods are still evolving; however, it appears that techniques of interviewing and examining possible victims are rapidly becoming more effective and more humane. Some communities already offer comprehensive evaluative services for sexual abuse (usually in a medical setting), and many others will develop them soon.

4.6.A Physical Abuse

Physical abuse is recognizable when there are signs of physical injury with discrepant explanations. In addition, there are some injuries that must be suspected as resulting from abuse and reported regardless of what history is given. Examples of the latter class are handmark bruises, fractures in healthy infants less than one year of age, hot water burns of the buttocks or burns of hands or feet in stocking or glove distribution, and linear marks on the skin resembling cord marks or belt marks. Examples of discrepant histories are the attribution of fractures to falls from beds (possible but rare) and the attribution of cigarette burns to insect bites.

Day care providers should identify physicians (who will usually be pediatricians) who are willing to provide them with telephone consultation about possible nonaccidental injury. This consultation should be used whenever a possible nonaccidental injury is discovered.

4.6.B Sexual Abuse

Most of the signs that young children may show when being sexually abused were listed in a preceding section (4.3.B). That many of these signs can also be produced by other causes presents a problem. A medical examination or a skillfully performed interview may be necessary in order to clarify the activities and participants.

One approach to this problem, which will help in many cases, is to ask the parent to seek professional help and to allow communication between the day care provider and the individual whom the parent consults. (It's a good idea to have a consent form for such communication signed by the parent or guardian, and to inform her or him when the form will be used.) Then, for example, a young child with a vaginal discharge may be referred to a physician who can determine if it is due to a yeast infection, which is not usually due to sexual abuse, or to gonorrhea, which is always associated with sexual abuse.[8]

Children who show behavioral symptoms of being sexually abused should be referred to professionals who are known to be skilled in the interpretation of such symptoms and in the techniques of play interview. Qualified individuals may be found among psychiatrists, psychologists, family counselors, social workers, and pediatricians. Some children will require both a medical and a behavioral examination. Finding professionals who are skilled in evaluating children for the possibility of sexual abuse may present some difficulties, but interest in this subject is widespread and the number of experienced persons is increasing rapidly. All professionals who work with children should acquire basic knowledge about child sexual abuse, and those who wish to perform special diagnostic work must prepare themselves appropriately. State Offices of Child Abuse Prevention and local child abuse councils are good sources of information about both training and consultation.

4.6.C Neglect

Because there are as many forms of neglect as there are of children's needs, and because mild neglect is difficult to separate from acceptable child-rearing practice, most states require that neglect, to be reported, should be producing some tangible harm. Some state laws include very specific diagnostic language, such as the term nonorganic failure to thrive, whereas others use general provisions. Day care providers should be prepared to recognize the possibility of neglect when certain signs are present, and, as with sexual abuse, many children will need a referral to a pediatrician.

Some instances of neglect may be perfectly obvious by the infant's or the child's appearance, the clothing provided, the state of hygiene, or the child's behavior. Others may be more subtle. Undernutrition is one common form of neglect that particularly affects infants less than two years of age. (Older children seem to be able to find food and eat it unless locked away from it.) Day care may well mask undernutrition because the infant makes up for the lack of food intake at home by feeding vigorously in care. Providers of care for infants need to be familiar with their normal appearance and patterns of linear growth and weight gain and to have some knowledge about normal intakes of food and formula.

Severe neglect of infants and children is likely to manifest itself as a developmental problem: either a general delay or specific areas of developmental lag. For example, delays in motor development occur in infants who are left in cribs with limited opportunity for movement; delays in speech occur in toddlers who are not spoken to. There are, of course, many other causes of these delays, but there is no question that the infant who is slow in any aspect of development must be thoroughly evaluated as soon as the fact is recognized. The pediatrician should generally be the professional person to start such an evaluation. The day care environment both treats and masks this type of problem, so it is likely to be more apparent when an infant is first brought for care.

4.6.D Alcohol and Substance Abuse

Alcohol or other chemical abuse by the parent is a very frequent factor in neglect or abuse of the infant. Dependency on drugs often allows many periods of relatively normal behavior by the parent which sometimes makes the problem difficult to recognize. A parent who is visibly intoxicated when he or she brings or picks up the child is, in most cases, addicted, but this event is relatively uncommon. It is much more common for a provider to notice that a parent smells of alcohol but is functioning pretty well. This circumstance should cause concern and should alert the provider to other manifestations of addiction. The question of alcoholism may also be raised when on frequent occasions the child is not brought for care and the parent doesn't go to work. Families whose lives appear chaotic despite apparent ability to function adequately in many social settings may well have an alcohol or drug problem in one or both parents.

Services for chemically dependent persons are numerous and accessible in most communities. The methods of intervention will vary in each case. If the problem has resulted in overt neglect or abuse of the child, the reporting laws apply as in any other case. Many persons with chemical dependency problems can be successfully treated, but initiating treatment is often very difficult. The pediatrician or the day care provider who suspects the problem and confronts the parent about it takes a high risk of being discharged. Confrontation is better done by another family member assisted by a person familiar with the treatment of chemical dependency. Care providers for the child should seek assistance from such sources.

4.7 Day Care as a Method for Prevention of Child Abuse

How much abuse has already been prevented by the use of day care can never be known, but the amount must be very large. Day care allows families to increase their incomes and to maintain higher standards of living than would otherwise be possible. Day care decreases isolation, and, for those parents who never experienced good care themselves, the providers of day care may be important models after whom they may pattern their own parental behaviors. Day care provides for reduction of the stress that can develop as a result of long periods of uninterrupted contact with infants or young children.

4.7.A Use of Day Care for Families at Risk for Abuse

Many families are perceived by professional persons as being very likely to abuse or neglect their children (see Appendix IV.2). Sometimes this is because they have already abused or neglected a child and have been referred to a protective agency. Sometimes it is because they manifest certain behaviors that often foreshadow or lead to child abuse or neglect. Such predisposing behaviors are often observed in the perinatal period and include such things as failure to seek prenatal care, use of alcohol or drugs, and making no preparation for the baby. Generational abuse, mental illness, family violence, and abuse of a prior child are also warning signals. After birth the same factors may be observed as well as impaired maternal-infant interactions, inappropriate discipline, unreasonable expectations of the infant, isolation, and near-abusive or mildly abusive actions. Premature birth is often associated with many of these behaviors, especially lack of prenatal care and failure to prepare for the baby, and premature infants as a group are much more likely to be abused or neglected than term babies.

Day care enriched, when possible, by special modeling or instruction is often sought by protective service workers for "high-risk" parents, and programs can be set up which emphasize this role.[9] For some parents such programs may provide the only exposure to healthy child-rearing practices that they have ever experienced. When day care providers are given special instruction about child abuse, they are more likely to become involved in prevention.[10]

Unfortunately, only a few day care providers are set up and funded as child abuse prevention services, and very few can afford to take the time that is required to bring about major change in the parenting practices of high-risk families. Services of this sort should be widely available but, in fact, they tend to be provided only in demonstration projects which cannot be replicated because of a lack of funding. Child care projects aimed at teenage mothers may be more common, and they serve the very useful purpose of allowing the young mother to complete her education while becoming attached to and caring for her infant with good models.[11] These programs may also prevent some abuse and neglect; however, it is not certain that the mothers that they reach are those most likely to abuse their children.

4.7.B Prevention of Sexual Abuse by the Education of Young Children

Educational programs which aim to "immunize" young children against being sexually abused have been developed in many places, and more appear every day.[12,13] Most such programs have quickly gained acceptance because of the public and professional concern about sexual abuse.

A typical program of this sort teaches children that they are allowed and empowered to say "NO!" or "STOP" when someone (anyone) touches them in a way which seems wrong or bad, and it teaches children about what is good and what is bad "touching." Instruction about how to escape and how to tell another trusted person about it is also given.

When programs of this sort are presented in schools, one effect is that some children will immediately tell the teacher that they are being sexually abused in their homes or in other places. Thus, a program aimed at preventing abuse initially results in dramatically increased reporting, which, in fact, actually does prevent the abuse from continuing.

Whether programs of this sort prevent sexual abuse is unknown and will remain so until some carefully designed and fairly long-term studies are performed. Even if they do, they are not ideal because they place the entire responsibility for the prevention of sexual abuse upon the child.[14] For the present, preschool educators should cautiously and carefully introduce such programs after consultation with skilled persons who work with sexually abused children.

4.7.C Educational Programs for Providers

The knowledge that educational programs about child abuse enhance the ability of providers to engage in prevention should encourage the development of this sort of instruction, both for persons in schools where child care and child development are taught and by organizations providing continuing education for active providers.

4.8 Implications

4.8.A Licensing

While day care licensing can probably never be a totally effective means for the prevention of abuse, it serves two important functions in limiting the amount of abuse that occurs. First, it makes possible easier interruption of abusive practices because removal of a license, which is a privilege, and not a right, requires a lower burden of proof than a criminal conviction for abuse. Second, a licensing review (whether or not it results in suspension) creates a record which may be valuable when the same person repeats the behavior on a later occasion. These two functions are important because child abuse is usually a private event for which documentation is often difficult, and determination of responsibility even more so. For casual, part-time child care providers, licensing could be a quick and simple process, but it would still make identification and checking of records possible.

4.8.B Education of the Public

Considerable effort should go into the preparation and dissemination of knowledge about day care and its relationships to child abuse. The many positive aspects should be mentioned along with the things that families can do to make their children safer. Pediatricians can assist in this process by having materials available in their offices and by covering the subject in the guidance they offer to parents.

References

1. Gelles RJ, Cornell CP: International perspectives on child abuse. *Child Abuse Negl* 1983;7:375-386
2. Kempe RS, Kempe DH: Incidence and Distribution of Sexual Abuse, in *The Common Secret: Sexual Abuse of Children and Adolescents*. New York, WH Freeman and Company, 1984
3. Kempe RS, Kempe CH: *Child Abuse*. Cambridge, MA, Harvard University Press, 1978, p 8
4. Martin HP: The consequences of being abused and neglected: How the child fares, in Kempe CH, Helfer RE, (eds): *The Battered Child*, ed 3. Chicago, The University of Chicago Press, 1980
5. Murray KA: Child care standards and monitoring, in Sharpe M (ed): *Daycare*. Report of the Sixteenth Ross Roundtable. Columbus, OH, Ross Laboratories, 1985, p 27

6. Summitt RC: The sexual abuse victim accommodation syndrome. *Child Abuse Negl* 1983;7:177-193
7. Blank H: Funding of Day Care and Public Policy, in Sharpe M (ed): *Daycare*. Report of the Sixteenth Ross Roundtable, Columbus, OH, Ross Laboratories, 1985, p 16
8. Sgroi S: Pediatric gonorrhea beyond infancy. *Pediatr Ann* 1979;8(5):73-87
9. Broadhurst D, Edmunds M, MacDicken RA: Early childhood programs and the prevention and treatment of child abuse and neglect. (For workers in Head Start, family day care, preschool and day care programs). Child Abuse and Neglect User Manual Series. DHEW Publication No. (OHDS), 79-30198. Washington, DC, US Government Printing Office, 1979, p 72
10. Barber-Madden R: Training day care program personnel in handling child abuse cases: Intervention and prevention outcomes. *Child Abuse Negl* 1983;7:25-32
11. Sung K-t: The role of day care for teenage mothers in a public school. *Child Care Quarterly* 1981;10:113-114
12. Anderson C, et al: Touch. (videotape: Illusion Theater, Minneapolis, Minnesota). Northbrook, IL, MTI Tele-Programs, Inc, 1980
13. Williams J, Softing K: *Red Flag, Green Flag People* (coloring book). Fargo, ND, Rape and Abuse Crisis Center of Fargo-Moorhead, 1980
14. Krugman RD: Preventing sexual abuse in day care: whose problem is it anyway? PEDIATRICS 1985;75:1150-1151

Chapter 5

PREVENTION, CONTROL, AND MANAGEMENT OF INFECTIONS IN DAY CARE

5.1 Introduction

Infections occurring in infants and children, adolescents, and young adults in various group settings have long been of concern to parents, physicians, and others in charge of their care. Staphylococcal and Group B Beta Streptococcal infections in newborn nurseries, Hepatitis A in group homes for the retarded, chicken pox and lice in public schools, poliomyelitis in summer camps, and meningococcal infections on military bases are among the most obvious examples.

With the increasing numbers of infants and children in day care, it is not surprising that considerable concern has arisen about infections in day care centers. Although controversy remains about the scope of this problem and the extent to which children in day care may be at increased risk for acquiring and spreading infections compared to children not in day care, there are certain basic principles concerning the control of the spread of infectious disease that must be strongly recommended. Of these, careful hand washing by personnel is the simplest and most important.

5.2 Personnel

5.2.A General Precautions

All personnel working in day care centers should have a medical evaluation and a tuberculin test prior to beginning work in the center and every two years thereafter. The examination is both for their own protection and to reduce the risk of their serving as a source of infection to the children (see

Appendix II.5). All personnel, including clerical, transportation, and food service workers, should be immunized according to the schedule recommended by the Centers for Disease Control (CDC) for caregivers in child care centers (Appendix V.1).

In large day care centers, workers should have a specific assignment within the center. If possible, food handlers should not also be caretakers, especially for infants and diaper-clad toddlers. Where personnel is limited by the size of the center, those handling infants and diaper-clad toddlers should not prepare food for others outside that group and should be especially meticulous about hand washing. Workers should care for the same children daily insofar as possible. This not only decreases the risk of spreading infections between groups of children, but provides the consistency of care desirable for the best development of the children.

Employees should maintain a high degree of personal cleanliness and should conform to good hygienic practices during all working periods. Staff members should thoroughly wash their hands and exposed portions of their arms with soap and warm water before starting to work, during work as often as necessary to keep them clean, after changing children's diapers or wiping their noses, and after smoking, eating, drinking, or using the toilet. Fingernails should be kept clean and should be trimmed. Outer clothing of all staff should be clean; and during the preparation and serving of food, effective hair restraints should be used to prevent contamination of food and food contact surfaces. Unsanitary practices such as scratching the head, placing fingers in or about the nose or mouth, or indiscriminate and uncovered sneezing or coughing without hand washing before returning to food preparation should be prohibited.

5.2.B Hand Washing

The most important measure in preventing the spread of infections in day care is hand washing. Personnel changing infants' and children's diapers and handling respiratory secretions (e.g., wiping a child's nose with a tissue) must conscientiously wash their hands and the children's hands after each such contact and after using the toilet themselves, using soap (liquid preferred) and running water. Hands should be rubbed vigorously as they are washed. The area washed should extend to the forearms. Thorough rinsing should be followed by drying the hands with a disposable towel which can then be used to turn off the faucets. Clean hands should not touch the bare faucet handles. A written reminder of the hand washing policy should be posted at each lavatory. Such reminders are frequently available from the local health department. Posters showing stepwise procedures for hand washing and diapering are available.

5.3 Medical Evaluation

All children should have a medical evaluation prior to entering into day care and their health should be monitored subsequently according to the schedule suggested by the American Academy of Pediatrics[1] (see Appendix V.2). Children in day care should be immunized as recommended by the Committee on Infectious Diseases of the American Academy of Pediatrics[2] (see Appendix V.3), and the history of their immunizations documented. The medical examiner should record preexisting infections which might be a risk to other children or day care workers, as well as conditions which might make the infant or child more likely to acquire infections. Children with significant immunodeficiency, whether congenital or acquired, should not be in group care. In large cities there may be programs developed exclusively for children with acquired immunodeficiency where specific precautions can be developed.

Children should be encouraged to learn and to practice good hygiene, especially in using the toilet, handling respiratory secretions, and feeding.

5.4 Facility

Day care centers should not be overcrowded. A written policy defining the maximum population should be developed, one that is consistent with the requirements of the children in care and with local or state health requirements and/or national consensus standards. In large centers, separate areas should be maintained for infants, diaper-clad toddlers, and toilet-trained toddlers. Ventilation should be adequate to minimize odors and dilute infectious agents. In general, the total ventilation area in every habitable room (one with operable windows) should not be less than 4.5% of the floor area, unless central air conditioning is provided.

Cleanliness is important. Floor surfaces and interior walls at the levels exposed to child contact should be easily cleanable. Such surfaces should be cleaned routinely according to a written schedule that complies with local or state health regulations or the orders of a pediatric consultant. Spot-cleaning of contaminated surfaces, such as infant seats and surfaces touched by the mouth, must take place before another child can use the equipment. Cleaning of all equipment should be done at least weekly. Visible soil should be removed daily. A sanitizing solution should be used after cleaning to rinse surfaces and toys in the infant and toddler areas before another child can use them. A solution which is inexpensive and effective can be made by adding ¼ cup of household bleach (5.25% sodium hypochlorite) to one gallon of water. This solution should be kept in a labeled container placed out of reach of the children and not near food or drink items. It must be made fresh daily, as it deteriorates rapidly, and the unused portions safely disposed of at the end of the day. The solution may be discarded in the sanitary sewer drain. A useful practice is to maintain a soap-and-water solution in a basin (out of reach of the children) into which contaminated toys are dropped until time permits washing, rinsing with the sanitizing dip, and air drying. Toys such as fuzzy stuffed animals, which cannot be adequately cleaned, should not be used in day care centers. There are machine-washable stuffed toys which are acceptable, but they should be treated as personal items. Children should be provided with separate receptacles for water play; most art materials also should not be shared but used by one child only and discarded when play is completed.

Sinks, lavatories, drinking fountains, and other water outlets should be supplied with safe water, sufficient in quantity and pressure to meet conditions of peak demand. The sewage or waste plumbing system should be designed, constructed, installed, and maintained to prevent cross-connection with the water system. Both plumbing and potable water systems should meet applicable standards of the local health department.

The center should provide at least one toilet and one lavatory located adjacent to the child care area for every 20 children or enough to prevent waiting. A center operating with children in attendance for five or more continuous hours a day should have as a minimum one toilet and one lavatory for every 15 children.

Toileting and diapering areas must be separate from the food preparation area. Potty chairs, when used, must be located only in a toilet area and must be wholly constructed of nonporous material. They should be dumped immediately, cleaned and sanitized prior to storage or reuse, either by using the chlorine solution specified for cleaning the toys and the diapering area or by using a commercial flusher designed for bedpan cleaning. Staff members should wear gloves while cleaning or sanitizing potty chairs. They should carefully wash their own hands when the procedure is completed. Sinks with hot and cold running water should be present in the toilet area and adjacent to the diaper-changing area. For safety, the hot-water temperature should not exceed 120°F at the outlet.

Sewage and other water-carried waste should be disposed of through a municipal sewer system when such a system is available. When a municipal system is not available, waste must be discharged into an approved private system which meets local health department requirements.

Garbage and refuse must be stored in fly-proof and water-tight containers with tight-fitting lids. Step-cans are preferable. A garbage can should be provided with a waterproof liner. Garbage and refuse ought to be removed from their containers and placed outside for collection or removal at regular intervals.

The premises should be maintained in a clean and sanitary fashion in order to prevent invasion by rodents and insects. A commercial exterminator should be called immediately if evidence of infestation is discovered. Under no circumstances should baits or other poisons be used in a way that presents a risk to the children.

5.5 Diapering Area

Caregivers should change children's diapers on disposable coverings, placed on a smooth, nonabsorbent, and easily cleaned surface, such as Formica or plastic. Dirty disposable diapers and table-coverings should be put immediately into plastic-bag-lined, foot-activated cans. Cans should be inaccessible to toddlers. Soiled clothing, including nondisposable diapers, should be placed immediately in separate plastic bags labeled with the child's name for individual laundering outside the center.

The diaper-changing area should be cleaned after every use with soap and water to remove visible soil, wiped with a sanitizing solution (see Section 5.4), and allowed to dry.

5.6 Food Preparation Area

When snacks and meals are provided by the day care center, the facility should comply with the sanitation requirements of the FDA Food Service Sanitation Manual (1976).[3] (Because there are so many sanitation issues involved in day care, a professional sanitarian should be employed to visit the facility to review practices and equipment even if not required by regulations to do so. Review should include food preparation, toilet, child care, and maintenance areas.)

At all times, while being stored, prepared, served, or transported, food should be protected from contamination by dust, insects, rodents, unclean equipment and utensils, unnecessary handling, coughs and sneezes, flooding, drainage, and overhead leakage or drippage from condensation. Containers of food should be stored a minimum of six inches off the floor in a manner that protects the food from splash. Potentially hazardous food (food capable of supporting growth of infectious or toxigenic microorganisms) should be refrigerated at 45°F or below or heated to 140°F or above. Foods should be stored in their original containers or in covered containers labeled as to contents.

Reusable equipment and utensils should be smooth, easily cleanable, corrosion-resistant or nonabsorbent, and durable under conditions of normal use. Nonporous material should be used for cutting boards, cutting blocks, salad bowls, and utensils. Single service articles should be made of clean, safe, and sanitary materials, and should not be reused.

To prevent cross-contamination, kitchenware and food contact surfaces should be washed, rinsed, and sanitized after each use and after any interruption of preparations during which contamination may have occurred. For manual washing, rinsing, and sanitizing of utensils, a commercial three-compartment sink is desirable. However, where only two compartments are available, a basin containing the sanitizing solution may be placed next to the sink. The third compartment, containing the sanitizing solution, should contain at least 50 parts per million of available chlorine (household bleach or other sanitizing solution) in the concentration specified by the local health department. The local health department can also advise regarding sources for sanitizer test-strips, to assure adequate concentration of the chlorine.

Mechanical dishwashers designed for home use are adequate for a day care facility. However, unless rinse temperatures reach 170°F for the period necessary to effect sanitation, the utensils should be rinsed in the aforementioned chlorine solution, or rinsed in hot water (170°F) for at least one-half minute.

Drain boards and racks of adequate size should be provided to allow the air drying of washed, rinsed, and sanitized utensils. Dish towels should not be used for drying utensils. Furthermore, sanitized instruments should not be drained on towels in place of a drain board or dish rack. Dried utensils should be stored in closed cabinets protected from dust, insects, rodents, and other sources of contamination.

Non-food-contact surfaces should be cleaned as often as necessary to keep the equipment free of accumulations of dust, dirt, food particles, and other debris. Cloths used for wiping spilled food on tableware, such as plates, bottles, and glasses, should be clean and used for no other purpose. Moist cloths or sponges used for wiping food spills on kitchenware and food contact surfaces should be cleaned and rinsed frequently in a sanitizing solution, such as the sanitizing solution of household bleach mentioned in Section 5.4. These cloths and sponges should be stored in the sanitizing solution between uses.

When a center provides infant formula, commercially prepared prebottled ready-to-feed formula should be used. Formula left in a bottle at the end of a feeding should be discarded. Commercial baby food containers that are opened, and foods prepared in the center which are stored, should be covered, dated, labeled as to the contents, and refrigerated. The contents should be discarded or used within a 36-hour period. A child should not be fed directly from baby food containers if the contents are to be fed to the child at more than one sitting or to more than one child.

When a parent chooses to provide formula or food, the center should assure that the food, formula, bottles, nipples, and containers comply with the following:

- Formula should be brought in a sealed container for terminal preparation just prior to feeding. Ready-to-feed formulas that are not commercially prebottled should be freshly bottled at the day care center from the can brought in unopened.
- Sanitized bottles may be provided by parents.
- Formula, breast milk, cow's milk, and perishable foods should be properly refrigerated.
- Foods and fluids must be covered and labeled as to contents, date of opening, and the child for whom they are intended.
- Formula should not be stored longer than 48 hours after opening.
- Foods other than formula should be used within 36 hours after opening or discarded.
- Milk brought in storage bottles to the center should be poured, just prior to use, into clean cups or bottles having sanitized nipples.
- Formula or milk left in a bottle or a cup at the end of a feeding should be discarded.

5.7 Sick Child Care

5.7.A Illness Policy

The center should have a written policy concerning the management of sick children. It should be conveyed in writing at the time a child is registered (see Appendix V.4). This policy, arrived at after consultation with health care providers, should take into consideration the physical facilities and the number and qualifications of the center's personnel. The decisions involved in developing policies are extremely difficult. It must be recognized that children do become ill at unpredictable times. Working parents often are not given leave for children's illnesses. Centers may not have sufficient space or personnel to care for sick children properly. Home care for sick children is expensive.

If an infant or child becomes ill during the hours he or she is in day care the parent(s) should be notified. To keep the infant or child in the child care program even temporarily, there must be adequate quiet space separate from the rest of the children where the sick child can be watched and given appropriate care. Staffing levels must be adequate to care for the sick child. Personnel must have sufficient training to recognize the child who requires prompt medical attention. Most states have laws requiring reporting of specific communicable diseases when they occur in a public facility. Child care personnel should be familiar with these requirements and promptly report the designated diseases. Day care staff members becoming ill with gastrointestinal or skin infections or who develop temperatures greater than 101°F should be excused from child care as quickly as possible. Sick leave policy should be as liberal as possible to prevent personnel from exposing children to infection.

5.7.B Exclusion Policy

There are very few illnesses for which children need to be excluded from day care. The center should identify, in its written policy, those diseases which require exclusion until the contagious stage is past. To facilitate decisions by both parents and staff, the policy should specify certain symptoms that make keeping a child away from the center advisable. Diarrhea, vomiting, specific types of rashes, and fever should be mentioned as well as such signs of illness as pallor, irritability, and excessive sleepiness. The specific list will depend on state laws, local public health recommendations, and suggestions made by the medical consultant for the day care program.[4,5,6] Programs which have staffing facilities to care for mildly ill children will be able to have more liberal policies than those with limited staffing and little space for ill children to receive the extra rest and supervision they require.

Deciding how to meet sick children's needs and parents' needs for child care is often difficult. Isolation and exclusion is not necessary for many illnesses. A balance must be struck between the needs of the child and the other children in the group and an arrangement made that does not strain the staffing resources of the day care program.

5.7.C Programs for Sick Child Care

There are a number of ways to provide care for sick preschool children. All methods include adequate rest, appropriate diet, giving medications as ordered, and physical and emotional support. A child can be cared for at home by a parent whose employer allows time off for the purpose. However, when care by the parent is not possible, a sick child may be accommodated in a variety of settings including:

- A separate area in the classroom
- A center shared by the day care center and the general community
- A freestanding center open to the public
- The child's own family day care home
- A freestanding family day care home serving only sick children
- A "satellite" home linked to a day care center or an agency
- The child's own home under supervision of an adult known to the parent(s), an employed caregiver, or a trained person from a home health agency or hospital.

5.7.D Disease Control

The spread of disease is prevented or minimized through precautionary measures that ought to be routine in day care programs. A detailed account of procedures used in managing specific diseases cannot be given here; the reader should consult the *Report of the Committee on Infectious Diseases* of the American Academy of Pediatrics for this kind of information.[1] Additional protocols for management of particular diseases can be found in references 4, 5, and 6.

The general recommendations that follow, intended for day care centers, are basic to good practice in minimizing the spread of specific types of infections within day care programs.[7]

1. *Infections spread by the fecal-oral route*

a. Enteric infections

The most common enteric infections encountered in the day care setting are hepatitis A, giardiasis, salmonellosis, and shigellosis.

Infants and children not yet toilet-trained are at the greatest risk of acquiring and transmitting these and other enteric infections spread by the fecal-oral route. Because of their young age and lack of previous exposure, they tend to be highly susceptible to the agents that cause them. Infants and young children mouth objects, wipe their noses with their hands, put hands in their diapers, and in their own and other children's mouths.

Objects given to infants such as teething rings and pacifiers should be used only for that child. They should be sanitized if dropped or otherwise contaminated. Community toys used by older children should also be sanitized if contaminated or visibly soiled.

It is imperative that those caring for children in diapers be aware of the risk of infection spreading to and from these children and take recommended precautions.

b. Pinworms

Pinworms are common in older infants and young children. The infestation is usually harmless. Children with rectal itching and girls with vaginitis due to pinworms should be treated. Although children who do not show symptoms can be examined and treated if infested, this is unnecessary and of little value, as parasites will inevitably be present in some children and not detected. Even if all children in the nursery are treated simultaneously, the pinworms will shortly thereafter be reintroduced. There is no reason to isolate children with pinworms or to notify families of "exposure," as all children in group settings can be assumed to be exposed to pinworms.

Careful attention to washing children's hands is the best

method of preventing the spread of pinworms and the reinfestation of the child from his/her own pinworms.

2. *Infections spread by the respiratory route*

Diseases included in this category include upper and lower respiratory tract infections due to viral agents and severe invasive diseases due to bacteria such as *Haemophilus influenzae* type b, and *Meningococcus*. These infections, if present in day care programs, can spread from asymptomatic carriers and from infected individuals who may or may not be symptomatic. Tuberculosis may spread from day care center personnel and other adults to children, but children with tuberculosis are not usually infectious because they do not produce infectious sputum.

Isolation of children with active respiratory infections has not been shown to be helpful in reducing the spread of airborne diseases in day care centers. However, careful hand washing by children and caregivers after direct contact with secretions and contaminated tissues may help to reduce the spread.

3. *Infections spread by direct contact*

a. Conjunctivitis

This inflammation of the conjunctivae is caused most commonly by a respiratory viral agent and sometimes by a bacterium, e.g., *H. influenzae*. It is contagious during the active infection and is spread through the watery or yellow eye discharge and by respiratory secretions. As with respiratory illnesses, careful hand washing by children and caregivers may help to reduce spread. Items like washcloths and towels, which may be contaminated by these effluvia, should not be shared.

b. Skin and hair infections

These include impetigo, scabies, lice, and ringworm. These infections are spread by person-to-person contact and by contact with contaminated objects such as combs, brushes, and towels. Basic hygienic measures, including avoidance of community towels, brushes, and combs, are important in reducing the spread of these infections in day care centers. Infected children should be appropriately treated. Exclusion of untreated children from the center should be considered.

4. *Diseases spread through urine, blood, saliva, and other bodily fluids*

This group includes such illnesses as herpes simplex

types 1 and 2, hepatitis B, cytomegalovirus (CMV), and acquired immune deficiency syndrome (AIDS). Herpes simplex type 1 virus is commonly shed in saliva by children with the diffuse lesions of acute herpetic gingivo-stomatitis, by those with more localized fever blisters, and, for various periods, by asymptomatic children. Children with acute herpetic gingivo-stomatitis are usually too ill to attend day care. Toys and items handled by children with fever blisters should be cleaned with the sanitizing solution. Caregivers handling these children do need to be careful about hand washing. Children with congenital herpes simplex type 2 may occasionally shed the virus when having recurrences of blisters. If these lesions are covered and caregivers are careful about hand washing after touching them, spread within the center should be prevented. Unlike hepatitis A, hepatitis B has not yet been shown to spread in day care centers. However, if a child who is a known hepatitis B carrier has an accident involving the spillage of blood, the blood should be carefully cleaned up with disinfectant solution. In addition, hepatitis B carriers should not share toothbrushes with other children (nor for that matter should any children). The risk in contacts is primarily one of acquiring infection from blood, and procedures to avoid contamination by blood from patients who are known type B carriers should be sufficient.

Children with congenital CMV infections may excrete virus in urine and saliva for long periods of time. However, normal asymptomatic children also frequently shed CMV in urine and saliva. Excretion of the virus by individuals both in day care centers and the general community is widespread. The concern has been expressed that pregnant women might acquire CMV from working in day care centers, thereby damaging their unborn children. Certainly, women of child-bearing age should be advised of this possibility. However, the risk cannot be avoided by excluding children with congenital CMV infections, since the excretion of the virus is widespread even in asymptomatic children. The emphasis instead should be on the importance of careful hand washing following contamination with urine and saliva.[8]

There is an ever-increasing amount of information available on which to base recommendations concerning the risks posed by children with AIDS attending day care centers. It is anticipated that both the Committee on Infectious Diseases of the American Academy of Pediatrics, and the Centers for Disease Control will continue to make statements concerning their management. For the present it is advisable to follow the recommendations in the *Report of the Committee on Infectious Diseases* of the American Academy of Pediatrics, Twentieth Edition.

5. *Infectious diseases preventable by vaccination*

Diphtheria, pertussis, tetanus, polio, measles, rubella, and mumps may be prevented by requiring immunization of all children attending day care. Immunization records should be kept on file and periodically reviewed to assure that the required immunizations for all children are up-to-date.

A new vaccine against *H. influenzae* type b has become available and should be given to children 2 to 5 years of age in day care centers[9] (see Appendix V.3). Varicella (chicken pox) vaccine will become available in the near future. Detailed recommendations concerning *Haemophilus* b polysaccharide vaccine (HBPV) can be found in the *Report of the Committee on Infectious Diseases* of the American Academy of Pediatrics, Twentieth Edition. Recommendations on varicella vaccine will be issued when the vaccine becomes available.

5.7.E Management of an Outbreak

When an infection spreads rapidly through a day care center despite routine precautions taken to prevent contagion, there should be a plan of action to manage the outbreak. The plan should be based on the care center as an entity, its designers having considered the interaction of all the individuals at the facility (adults as well as children) and the points at which communication of the etiologic agent can be most effectively interrupted. Outside sources should be contacted promptly for professional guidance in current measures of control. Medical advice and service will be necessary for the institution of appropriate therapy and possibly for diagnostic tests to confirm infection or to discover it in asymptomatic individuals.

If containment of the outbreak (or the physical condition of the child) requires exclusion from the day care program, alternate care arrangements should be implemented in accordance with exclusion policies already established (see section 5.7.B). It must be emphasized that decisions concerning exclusion, alternate care, and readmission will be easier to make if plans are in place when the need for them arises. It is helpful, also, if the day care center has gathered information in advance concerning sources to cover or assist with payment for diagnosis, treatment, and alternative care. Plans that specify services that parents (or the day care center) cannot afford are not practical.

The array of precautionary measures necessary to maintain the health of children in group care may seem overwhelming to day care administrators or staff members who have asked advice of the health consultant in designing their program. The consultant must be aware that in many instances his or her work is not complete when all the rules have been laid out; to be effective, the health professional has to convince care providers that health maintenance procedures are indeed practical, that once in place they become second nature to a well-trained staff, and that, above all, they are very, very important.

References

1. Committee on Infectious Diseases: *Report of the Committee on Infectious Diseases*, ed 19. Evanston, IL, American Academy of Pediatrics, 1982
2. Committee on Infectious Diseases: California Chapter No. I, American Academy of Pediatrics: *Infections in Day Care Centers: Recommendations for Prevention and Control.* 1984 (unpublished)
3. A model food service sanitation ordinance. US Department of Health, Education and Welfare, DHEW Publication # (FDA) 78-208, Public Health Service. Food and Drug Administration, Division of Food Service, Washington, DC, 1976

4. Minneapolis Health Department: *Infectious Diseases in Child Day Care: Information for Day Care Center Directors and Parents or Guardians.* Minneapolis, MN, Minnesota Department of Health, 1983
5. Mecklinburg County Health Department: *Report on Child Day Care.* Charlotte, NC, Mecklinburg County Health Department, 1983
6. Mecklinburg County Health Department: *Protocol for Management of Infections in Child Day Care Facilities.* Charlotte, NC, 1983
7. Bartlett AV, Broome CV, Hadler SC, et al: Public health considerations of infectious diseases in child day care centers. *J Pediatr,* 1984;105:683-701
8. Pass RF, Kinney JS: Child care workers and children with congenital cytomegalovirus infection. PEDIATRICS 1985;75:971-973
9. Committee on Infectious Diseases: *Haemophilus influenza* type b polysaccharide vaccine. PEDIATRICS 1985;76:322-323

Bibliography

Michigan Department of Public Health: *Communicable Disease in Child Care Settings,* 1985
Child Welfare League of America: *Standards for Day Care Services,* revised. New York, Child Welfare League of America, 1984
Seattle-King County Department of Public Health: *Day Care Health Program.* Seattle, WA, Seattle-King County Department of Public Health, 1985

Chapter 6

PREVENTION, CONTROL, AND MANAGEMENT OF INJURIES IN DAY CARE

6.1 Introduction

Injuries do not just happen; the majority are predictable and preventable. Because child care settings share some attributes of home and school environments, many of the injury control measures which are effective in homes and schools are directly applicable to child care facilities. Information about hazards which are a significant cause of injury to children in the general population is available from the National Electronic Injury Surveillance Systems (NEISS) of the U.S. Consumer Product Safety Commission (USCPSC). NEISS collects injury data from a statistically representative sample of U.S. hospital emergency rooms. The data are ranked by the product involved in the injury and by the frequency and severity of injury. Studies of injury-related factors conducted by the USCPSC suggest procedures that are likely to reduce injuries. These measures are generally useful in preventing injuries caused by a faulty product or part of the environment within day care facilities.

Unfortunately, there are no national data on the incidence of injury in day care programs specifically, although the National Safety Council does collect such data for schools. One study of insurance claims from child care programs suggested some special considerations which deserve emphasis for injury control in the child care setting.[1] This study found that nearly two thirds of injuries which were severe enough to require medical attention occurred on the playground. Playground equipment, especially climbers and to a lesser extent, swings, were most commonly associated with the most severe injuries. Hand toys, blocks, doors, and indoor floor surfaces also ranked high on the list of products which were associated with more frequent and more severe injuries. Because of these associations, specific recommendations about injury control related to these parts of a child care facility are made in this chapter. For additional information on injury control, consult the Academy's handbook on *Injury Control for Children and Youth,*[2] or contact the USCPSC and the National Safety Council (see Appendix VI.1 for addresses).

Injury control requires consideration of the physical plant (facility and equipment) as well as program policies and procedures which govern human action in the child care environment. One procedure helpful in identifying hazards in the physical plant is the use of routine periodic safety inspections. Parents, staff, and children can share in this activity. A checklist keyed to each part of a center's facility will remind the inspectors to check potential causes of trouble. A "safety walk" using such a checklist is an educational experience for all participants. By rotating the responsibility for safety surveys among the personnel, hazards invisible to one pair of eyes will be discovered by another and everyone's awareness of safety and environmental quality will be heightened. A sample safety checklist can be found in Appendix VI.2.

Hazard reduction need not be expensive or difficult. Sometimes the provision of adequate storage, relocation of a handrail, changing the placement of furniture, or covering sharp edges is all that is required to reduce the risk of injury. Institution of simple safety measures in the child care center has the added benefit of showing ways to make home environments safe for children.

6.2 Environmental Safety

6.2.A Prevention of Injury in Active Play

Playgrounds are used by children to release pent-up energy and by caregivers to find relief from confinement. Tempering these pleasant associations is the fact that gross motor play areas, especially playgrounds, are the sites of greatest risk of injury in child care. Playground equipment is ranked high on the U.S. Consumer Product Safety Commission's list of the top ten products associated with significant injury in the pediatric age group.

The Commission's studies have found that over 70% of the injuries on play equipment are the result of falls.[3] Injuries occur because of pushing, shoving, dare-devil behavior, inattention, unanticipated use of equipment, crowding, and simultaneous use of equipment by children of different ages. Poor play area design, resulting in lack of control of traffic flow around equipment, also contributes to injuries.

Many types of equipment used for gross motor play have elevated surfaces that lack adequate barriers to prevent falls. Workplace standards of the Occupational Safety and Health Administration (OSHA) require installation of a double guard rail to protect adult workers in areas raised four feet or more above the floor (about two thirds of adult height).[4] Many structures for climbing used by preschool children are more than twice their height and yet lack guard rails. Based on USCPSC guidelines, all elevated surfaces which might be climbed and which are more than 30 inches above the underlying surface should have protective barriers at least 38 inches in height completely surrounding the elevated surface, except for entrance and exit openings.[5] Climbers and slides used by preschool and younger children should be limited to six feet at the highest point and protected at the entrance and exit to prevent falls. Metal climbers and slide beds should be located away from direct sun since they quickly overheat in sunny locations.

Since falls to a surface are a common source of injury, it is appropriate to look at ways to reduce the damage that they cause. A study reported in 1979 by the National Bureau of Standards[6] indicated that even low velocity falls onto asphalt or concrete will produce concussions and other injuries. However, results of impact testing indicated that surfaces composed of six inches or more of loose materials such as pine bark or shredded tires meet the impact-attenuation criterion recommended for drop-heights of up to ten feet. Tested unitary materials such as rubber mats and synthetic turf do not meet the criterion beyond five feet. The shock-absorbing capacity of loose materials decreases with repeated impact because the materials consolidate, essentially reducing the thickness. Thus, to maintain the cushioning effect of loose fill materials, continuous care is required. Using thicker layers than those tested reduces the need for frequent maintenance.

No playground surfacing material is perfect. Sand becomes cohesive when wet, therefore less cushioning; in freezing temperatures, it offers no cushioning protection at all. Both sand and builders' round stone (pea gravel) can be thrown into eyes; all loose fill materials harbor and conceal foreign materials such as insects, animal excrement, broken glass, nails, and other injurious objects. Pine bark mininuggets and various mulch materials absorb moisture and become compact, losing some of their cushioning properties. Over time, they decompose, providing a medium for growth of molds and microorganisms. Like sand, they can freeze solid in cold weather. When wet, these materials tend to stain clothing. Shredded tire rubber and crushed stone (blue stone dust) have some advantages over materials which decompose but pose the same problem of concealing hazardous objects. Thus, loose fill materials must be hosed down for cleaning and require raking for removal of hazardous objects and leveling to maintain effective cushioning depth. Asphalt and cement are the worst surfaces to have under climbers; soil or grass are also poor surfaces compared to loose fill material.

Safe areas for young children to climb on can be planned to provide heights by using mounds or hills rather than elevated platforms or bars over hard surfaces. Slides can be built into mounds to reduce the risk of falls. Equipment designed for older children can be removed from areas where younger children usually play. Regardless of design, play equipment must be maintained in good repair. There should be no pinch- or crush-points, no exposed screws and bolts, no sharp edges, no rings which permit head entrapment, no hard, heavy swing seats, no open or "S" hooks, loose nuts, or splinters. All steps and rungs intended for foot placement should be horizontal and at least 15 inches wide; hand grips should be no larger than 1.6 inches in diameter to permit firm holding. Every climbing surface should include handrails or hand grips.

Outdoor play areas should be fenced whenever possible because of the risk of mixing the activities of play with street traffic, thoughtless passers-by, and unrestrained pets. However, the view of all parts of the playground must not be obstructed. Even with fencing, maintenance will be required to keep the play area free of broken glass, stagnant water, animal excrement, holes, trash, and litter. Shaded areas should be provided, but care must be taken to avoid planting bushes, shrubs, or trees that produce toxic berries, leaves, or stems. All water-play areas should be fenced. Gates should be kept locked.

Other playground measures will also reduce risk of injury. There should be clearly marked danger zones to prevent children from walking into the path of swing seats or exits from slides. Children should be segregated by developmental stage for play on gross motor apparatus to prevent younger children from being injured by imitating or encroaching on the more skillful play of older children. Wherever possible, barriers can be used to prevent collisions of playing children. Detailed technical guidelines governing construction, location, and installation of gross motor play equipment and surfacing are available from the USCPSC.[3,5]

It is not possible to create a totally safe playground because some degree of risk taking is an important ingredient of play. Children have to learn how to play safely, just as the adults who supervise them have to learn how to minimize potential injury. Many child care planners overlook opportunities to involve children in learning about safe play. There are safety principles for children to learn for each type of equipment. For example, for swings: sit in the center, never stand or kneel; stop the swing before getting off; walk 'way around the swing; never push anyone else on the swing or allow another child to push you; one person on the swing at a time; empty swings should not be swung; swing-chairs must always be straight, never twisted, etc.

Not all injuries in active play areas can be prevented, but monitoring of injury reports in this area, as in the rest of the facility, can provide clues about possible corrective measures. Supervision should be planned by establishing a written schedule, and assigning more staff to areas of high risk (e.g., near climbing structures, slides, and swings). Making benches or other comfortable seats available near high-risk areas encourages adults to stay nearby. Active playtime is not adult break time.

6.2.B Prevention of Injuries from Hazards in the Facility

Safety surveillance and supervision of areas of high risk

are advisable everywhere in the facility. The safety of employees who work in day care facilities that are not directly government operated is protected under the Occupational Safety and Health Act, administered by the Occupational Safety and Health Administration (OSHA) of the U.S. Department of Labor. OSHA provides a free on-site consultation service in every state. Consultants help identify hazardous conditions and suggest corrective measures in a written report. The consultation is confidential, provided only on request, separate from an inspection, and no citations are issued. By use of the service, hazards for both adults and children can be detected and corrected. (See Appendix VI.3 for OSHA Consultation Service Project Directory.) Other sources of assistance for risk reduction are the fire department, local poison control centers, public health departments, Red Cross chapters, hospitals, medical schools, insurance agencies, and local/regional offices of the U.S. Department of Housing and Urban Development (HUD). Hazards in day care facilities can be corrected to minimize accidents, including those that are associated with fires. (Although some fire safety measures for day care are mentioned below, an updated, comprehensive guideline for day care centers, group homes, and family day care homes can be found in the Life Safety Code of the National Fire Protection Association.[7]) Safety can be enhanced if the following precautions are taken:

1. Stairways are known to be safer when they are well illuminated and equipped with handrails on the right side descending. Light switches should be accessible at each entry to a room in the facility. Because stairways are likely places for injury, supervision of stairway use should be planned as for the playground. Children need to learn to ascend and descend stairs carefully, holding onto the handrail. Adults who set good examples help.

2. Stairways and stairwells should not be used as storage areas.

3. All exterior or interior doors that open onto a stairway should have a gate or landing. Doors need devices that prevent rapid closure, vision panels down to child level, safety glass or plexiglass panels, (with opaque marks on large clear panels to make them visible), and beveled edges to prevent crushed fingers. All stairwells, elevated walkways, elevated porches, and elevated play areas ac-

cessible to children should have railings or adaptations to prevent falls. Openings from high places that are large enough to permit the passage of a child's body should be closed inexpensively by weaving rope across the space, using screw eyes at the edges of the opening. The netting achieved should be closely woven to prevent head entrapment.

4. All windows above the ground floor that are accessible to preschool children should be constructed, adjusted, or adapted with window stops, screens, or grills to limit their opening to less than six inches.

In the event of a collision of sufficient force to break a glass pane, the victim is subject to injury which may be severe. Windows that are in the path of play should be safety glazed, replaced by plexiglass, or protected from breakage by guards. Sill heights that are at least 12 inches above the floor help prevent such collisions.

5. Floors should be made safe by removing trip hazards and by breaking up long runways with furniture or equipment to discourage running. Basements in old buildings may have floors with rough surfaces and deep pits. The hazard is increased by poor lighting. These areas should be filled and leveled. Properly installed and padded carpet offers the best slip resistance and sound control for flooring in day care. The grade and fabric content should be suited to frequent cleaning. Carpeting should not be used where contamination by food, secretions, or excrement is likely, however. In such areas, slip-resistant tile or slip-resistant coated nonporous floor materials should be used.

6. Lockable enclosures used by children should be designed to permit adults to enter in case of emergency.

7. All hallways should be wide enough for two adults.

8. Exit routes should be unobstructed. Exit doors should have a panic bar and only one locking or latching device.

9. All clear glass panels in traffic areas should be made of safety glass or its equivalent and marked to reduce the likelihood of accidental impact.

10. All heaters, furnace registers, hot water pipes, tap water, and other sources of heat accessible to children should not exceed 110°F at the point of access, to prevent burns. Wrapping, insulation, and partitions can be used to prevent contact with pipes, registers, and radiators. If poten-

tially hazardous asbestos is thought to be present in the insulation, the site should be inspected by the local or state-designated agency. If present and in poor or only fair condition, it should be removed and other materials substituted. Thermoregulated mixing valves can be inexpensively installed in the hot water supply that leads to children's sinks when the main water heater cannot be turned down because of hot water requirements for dishwashing equipment. At least two feet, six inches of clear space should be allowed in front of all heating and air conditioning units.[8]

11. Heating equipment should be enclosed in fire-resistant material installed and maintained consistent with the current standards of the National Fire Protection Association.[7]

12. All equipment should be checked for conformity to recommended safety standards. Standards for infant furniture and playground equipment are available from USCPSC. Another helpful source is the American Society for Testing and Materials from which copies of specific standards may be ordered (see Appendix VI.1 for addresses).

    a. There should be no loose or frayed electric wires in the facility.

    b. Electric equipment must not require the use of long extension cords or be situated near water; overloading of sockets should be avoided. Nonmetallic, tight-fitting caps should be inserted into electric receptacles that are not in service in areas where young children are in care. In new construction, receptacles can be located above the reach of small children.

    c. Free-standing space heaters should not be used: besides burns, they may cause air pollution resulting in respiratory disease.

    d. All fans should have covers or guards with openings smaller than one half inch.

    e. Aerosol cans should be inaccessible to children and stored away from any heat source.

13. There should be no poisonous plants in a child care facility or accessible to any area where children play. (See Appendix VI.4 for a list of poisonous plants.)

14. Since many day care programs are located in older buildings, the paint on walls and woodwork should be checked for lead content. Blistered or chipped old paint may be-

come paint dust on the floor and accessible to children who put nonedibles in their mouths. This is particularly important for family day care homes in geographic areas known to have lead paint problems.

15. Medications and cleaning solutions should be kept in their original containers, with safety lock closures. Storage areas should be made inaccessible to children by using special latches or other safety devices.

16. Toxic art materials should not be used. Craft objects which are small enough to lodge in ears or noses must be available only where close supervision is possible. (See Appendix VI.5 for a list of unsafe art supplies.)

17. Activities known to be associated with frequent injury require close supervision. It is important that equipment and materials are used as intended. Since blocks are a problem when the children use them as hammers and balls, staff members should set strict rules about behavior and stay nearby to enforce them. Control of the number of children using potentially troublesome toys at any time may also help.

18. Toys should be regularly inspected and maintained. Broken toys should be placed out of service until fixed or discarded. Propellant toys are not safe because of potential eye injuries and aspiration or ingestion of propelled objects.

19. Styrofoam cups and brittle plastic forks are choking hazards because small pieces may easily break off when these objects are chewed.

20. Cooking utensils and equipment used in educational activities should be carefully selected to avoid risk of injury to children. Electric frying pans are commonly used in day care for out-of-kitchen projects. They are especially dangerous because they give no sign to show when they are hot.

6.2.C Transportation Safety

6.2.C.1 Passenger Safety

Through efforts initiated by the American Academy of

Pediatrics during the International Year of the Child, there are now laws in most states requiring that very young children be transported in child safety seats. These laws vary from one state to another, covering children of different ages, affecting some or all drivers, and requiring restraints in different seating positions. In some states, regulations or laws specifically require that child care programs use child safety seats or seat belts when such devices are available in the vehicle. By 1981, the National Highway Traffic Safety Administration found that safety seat usage had increased to 46.1% for children under five years of age.[9] Unfortunately, even though safety seat use has significantly increased, 65% of the seats are being used incorrectly.[10] There is still much work to be done. Although the legal requirements only affect the youngest children, *no child of any age* (or adult for that matter) *should be exposed to the risk of motor vehicle travel without the protection of an appropriate seat restraint.*

Child care personnel have three roles to play in reducing the toll taken by vehicular accidents, the number one killer of children:

1. As advocates of safe transport of children by their parents and others
2. As safe transporters of children
3. As educators of young children about how to be safe riders

Each of these roles provides an opportunity for integration of child passenger safety with other activities that are accepted parts of the child care program.

At the very least, child care personnel have a responsibility as informed child advocates to assure that parents transport their children safely on every ride. Since 1981, all child safety seats manufactured in the United States have had to meet the federal requirement that the seats stand up to crash forces if used according to the manufacturer's instructions. To be effective, the seat must not only be appropriate for the age and size of the child, but it must also be used correctly. Common errors in car seat use are: 1) failure to use a required harness; 2) failure to secure the seat properly with the car's lap belt; and 3) failure to use a properly mounted tether strap when one is required. Worst of all is allowing a child to ride unrestrained in a vehicle in which a child safety device is available. Detailed information on car seats and their proper use is available through the Every Ride A Safe

Ride Program of the American Academy of Pediatrics. Most state chapters of the AAP have an Every Ride Coordinator. In addition, the national office of the AAP can provide child passenger safety information.

Booster seats and shields are favored by day care administrators because they are inexpensive, light-weight, adaptable to the widest range of child sizes (usually 20 to 55 or 60 pounds), and take up the least amount of room in a vehicle. Most booster and toddler seats increase the child's ability to see out the vehicle windows and are designed for use until the child grows big enough to look out without the device. Children who can watch through the windows behave better while they ride, and that fact is a good selling point for use of car seats to both parents and caregivers.

For the child over four years of age or weighing more than 40 pounds, a regular seat belt can be used. There is no evidence that using an adult shoulder harness for a child results in increased injury. As long as the strap does not actually cross the child's face and can be adjusted for comfort over the neck, the shoulder portion of a belt should always be used. The safest place for anyone to ride is in the rear seating position, but seat belts or car safety seats should be used in all seating positions. Some states permit the use of lap belts for very young children; however, this measure is a compromise to be used only when a properly designed, correctly installed child safety seat is unavailable. Parents should be told repeatedly that it is always better for children to ride restrained than loose.

Child care programs almost always involve transportation in some way. As a minimum, parents bring children to and from the day care facility daily. This provides an ideal opportunity to observe whether parents are using child safety seats or seat belts and whether they are using them correctly. Part of the orientation procedure for new families should include a review of transportation arrangements and the provision of a checklist of safe ride pointers. On the first day the children attend the program, a staff member should be available to check whether they are arriving and leaving safely restrained. Some parents may require demonstrations and gentle instruction to correct unsafe practices.

Child care personnel are responsible for making sure that the drop-off and pick-up points are large enough and sheltered from street traffic so that parents are protected as they buckle and unbuckle their children and carry or walk them from the car to the program building. Staff should routinely be stationed in a location that permits them to help during arrival and departure times; extra hands may be needed to take children out of their seat restraints, safely secure them, or escort them to and from vehicles.

When parents use car pools to move children between home and child care centers, there are special concerns. All the drivers must be known to be responsible and willing to assure that every one regularly buckles up. There should be rules for car capacity, discipline, and use of safety restraints. No car should ever carry more passengers than there are seat restraints. The risk far exceeds the convenience. There should be policies for driver substitution. The procedures used for drop-off and pick-up must be clearly spelled out in advance and should provide for the increased time and supervision required to buckle and unbuckle the number of children involved. All parents need adequate liability insurance coverage and must agree to assume responsibility for regular auto maintenance checks on tires, brakes, and steering systems.

Some state laws or regulations provide additional incentives for compliance with transportation safety procedures. Some specify requirements for drivers. Check to see what is required. Even if state law does not cover all drivers or if day care regulations are not specific about it, all day care drivers should be required to have preservice training in routine safety and emergency procedures. Remind drivers that failure to buckle up children poses an unacceptable risk and could expose the driver to being sued if a child is hurt. Plan driving routes to minimize backing up (to prevent backing over children who run behind the car), and to avoid hazardous turns and dangerous intersections. On every trip, enough time must be allowed in the schedule to eliminate the pressure of loading, unloading, or driving when late.

To make trips as safe as possible, parents or drivers they employ should:

1. Pick up and discharge children only at the curb.
2. Have other parents put their own children with their safety seat into the car and buckle them up; let parents take the children out of the car on the return home.
3. Place all hard objects, such as lunch boxes or things for show and tell, on the floor.
4. Close and lock all car doors after checking that all fingers

and feet are inside. Auto dealers sell inexpensive safety locks that keep little hands from opening doors but are no barrier to an adult.

5. Open passenger windows only a few inches. Turn off power window controls except at the driver's location.

6. Remind the children about the rules of behavior before starting to drive. Point out interesting things the children can see to make the trip a positive experience and include them in pleasant conversation. Bored children are more likely to try to get out of their safety seats or make trouble for the other children. Plan simple games or songs for the trip such as "Who can find a stop sign? a red light? a green light? a truck? a blue car?" There are many songs like "The Wheels of the Bus Go 'Round" which help make the trip less tedious. Praise the children often for appropriate behavior.

7. Plan transportation routes realistically to keep travel time down to the tolerance of the riders. No child should have to be in the vehicle more than an hour.

8. Find a safe place to pull over, if any child or the group gets out of hand, before trying to discipline anyone. Be firm, state the rules clearly, and praise good behavior. If any child is a problem consistently, exclude the child from group transport unless special arrangements are made.

9. Identify children whose special characteristics (behavior, age, disability) require special arrangements and plan for them.

10. Be sure each vehicle is equipped with a fire extinguisher, first aid kit, emergency identification, and contact information for all children being transported.

When transportation is a service of the child care program, staff members must observe the same safety rules as parents. Additionally, the program administrators must address issues related to liability insurance, training, and certification of drivers, first aid supplies and emergency equipment, ready access to emergency help and medical information in the event of an accident, proper equipment and labeling of vehicles, and permission slips for whatever purpose transportation is being used. Large groups from a child care center can be accommodated in school buses. However, the safety features of school buses are specifically designed for use by school-aged children. Buses made after 1977 can be equipped with seat belts for safe transport of young children. The cost for this type of installation ranges between $10 and $30 per belt. Vans often come equipped with lap belts which make it possible to use child safety seats. If seats that require harnesses are used, the harness tethers must be properly installed. Vehicles cannot be used to transport more children than can be *safely buckled up.*

Teaching passenger safety to young children is important. Children must learn to ride only with drivers they know and only buckled up. Children can learn how to buckle themselves into their safety seats very early and to insist that not only they, but all the riders in the vehicle, are buckled up.

Safe polite riding can be taught with games, flannel boards, songs, stories, and all the other methods familiar to early childhood educators. A good example of suitable preschool literature is the 1983 publication "When I Ride in a Car" by Dorothy Chlad (Children's Press, 1224 West Van Buren St., Chicago, IL 60607, $6.95). A curriculum package developed for the National Highway Safety Administration is quite useful; information about other early childhood curricular materials is available through the National Association for the Education of Young Children (see Appendix VI.1 for address). To make safety props for classroom play, visit a junk yard with a sturdy pair of scissors and cut off seat belts to mount on classroom chairs for safe "pretend" rides. To obtain car safety seats for the classroom, seek donations from families whose children have outgrown them.

Some child care centers have developed car seat "loaner" programs for parents. This is an undertaking that requires considerable effort, but is a valuable alternative to bake sales for parent involvement. Several of the car seat manufacturers and many of the child passenger safety organizations will provide free instructions to start up and run a car seat loaner program.

6.2.C.2 *Pedestrian Safety*

Streets in the vicinity of child care facilities can be marked by "Children at Play" or similarly worded signs provided by local police or highway departments. Walking trips should be planned in advance to identify safe routes and to establish procedures to cross intersections safely. Reading material on pedestrian safety that is suitable for young children is available from local chapters of the American Automobile Association.

6.2.D Swimming

Swimming activities are a worthwhile learning experience for young children but one that requires adequate staffing, staff training, and appropriate facilities. Pools should meet requirements for public bathing facilities. In most states these requirements should include training of supervisory staff, frequent inspection of equipment, and routine checks on the water quality by pool staff and health inspectors. All bodies of water located where children can have access to them should be restricted by enclosures with a locked gate. Portable wading pools are acceptable if only one child uses the pool and the pool is emptied and cleaned after each use. Even with filtration and chlorination systems, a wading pool functions simultaneously as a communal toilet and giant drinking cup for young children. Unless a portable pool is used as an outdoor bathtub for one person, it provides a superior means of transmission of infectious diseases.

For swimming activities the ratio of staff members to children should be at least double that normally required for the age and group size, and the staff should include individuals with competence, and preferably with certification in advanced water safety and cardiopulmonary resuscitation techniques. All staff, volunteers, and other adults who are counted in the adult-child ratio for swimming activities should have successfully completed basic water safety instruction from a certified water safety instructor.

6.2.E Guns

Children are naturally curious about all objects in their environment. Guns are kept by adults for many reasons, including recreational use and self-defense. The risk of a gun accident involving a child must be weighed against the reason for the gun to be kept at all. Many fatalities have occurred because of children having easy access to a gun. Other security systems such as alarms are far preferable.

However, day care programs are located in homes and in areas where adults may keep guns. If guns are permitted, strict rules are needed to prevent children from gaining access to these weapons and the equipment associated with them. Such rules include:

- No loaded gun should be permitted in a child care facility.
- Store ammunition in a locked enclosure separate from the location of the gun.
- Secure the gun with a trigger lock that can be removed only by using a special key or wrench. The wrench or key should be locked up separately.
- Remove the firing pin from souvenir guns.

6.3 Emergency Preparedness

6.3.A Disaster Planning

Planning for evacuation in the event of fire, flood, tornado, sudden loss of heat or air conditioning, or other disaster is essential. Fire emergency plans should include use of direct and alternative exit routes and practice of evacuation drills at different times of the day, including nap time. Drills should be held at least once a month. An alternative shelter should be arranged to which the children can be taken and parents informed of it in advance. Daily attendance records and the information necessary to reach parents must be maintained in a portable fashion so that these files can be removed with the children and staff as a part of the evacuation procedure.

Assignment and instruction of staff members should ensure safe evacuation of all the children to a prearranged location inside or outside the facility within two minutes of an unannounced alarm. The chain of command and duties of staff members are best worked out in advance so that it is clear who will verify that the evacuation is complete, who will notify the rescue or fire authorities, who will contact the parents, and how the security of the facility will be handled.

Fire extinguishers in working order should be available and staff members should know how to use them. Fire alarms should be conspicuous and unobstructed. Emergency lights must be functional and located so that exit routes are illuminated in an emergency.

The standards of the National Fire Protection Association Life Safety Code appropriate to the type of facility should be applied by a qualified building or fire inspector to assure identification of correctable hazards. Inspectors can be very helpful, not only in identifying problems, but in suggesting solutions and informing program administrators of resources to implement the solutions. Evaluation of heating systems, electric wiring and appliances, and cooking equipment hazards requires technical competence that is often outside the province of child care personnel.

6.3.B Individual Emergencies

No matter how safety conscious the staff members and children become, some injuries will occur. Most will be minor, requiring simple first aid and no professional medical attention. Because the principles of first aid are easily learned by caregivers and children, these measures should be included in staff training and the child care curriculum. Extensive, formal first aid training courses are not necessary, since they often emphasize survival skills that exceed the requirements of most day care settings. However, the special first aid approaches that are appropriate for children should be taught by a competent health professional. (See Appendix VI.6 for a sample set of first aid instructions for child care program use.)

Staff members should be able to reach parents (or persons specified by the parents) at any time to report an emergency. The child care center should have on file the names and telephone numbers (at home and at work) of individuals responsible for each child. It is a good idea for day care personnel to verify the emergency contact person's availability and willingness to serve by trying to call the telephone numbers provided. Emergency information should also include the name and telephone number of the child's usual source of health care. Because these facts change from time to time, it is important to update the records periodically, at least every six months. When an emergency occurs, all of this information should be easily accessible. If trips away from the day care facility are taken or transportation is provided, emergency information must be with the adult who is responsible for the children.

Emergencies are best handled when there is a clear chain of command: someone must call for transport to a source of emergency medical care; someone must notify the parents; someone must accompany the child; someone must attend to the needs of the other children in the group who witnessed the child's injury. The caregiver or designated adult who is responsible for the child must be able to stay with the child until the parents arrive to take over. Parents cannot give informed consent in advance for medical care in emergency situations because the nature of the medical care that might be required is not known. Although many doctors and hospitals provide care without parental consent, they are not protected legally unless the situation is life-threatening. Parents should be informed when the child is enrolled that their whereabouts must be known at all times.

The prevention, control, and management of injuries in day care is based on careful planning and continual updating of procedures and contact information. When an accident happens, often much can be learned about prevention from the way in which the accident occurred and the way it is handled. Injury reports should be filed in a central location as well as in the child's record (see Appendix VI.7). Periodic review of the reports will reveal incidents that occur repeatedly and must be prevented by modification of the facility or procedures. Staff and parent responses to emergency situations should be reviewed to reveal deficiencies that require more training and information to be eliminated. Expert help from the community may be necessary to assist with planning, training, or correction of hazardous situations. Physicians, nurses, public health authorities, and fire safety and civil defense personnel should be willing to act as consultants.

References

1. Aronson SS: Injuries in child care. *Young Children* 1983;38:19-20
2. Committee on Accident and Poison Prevention: *Injury Control for Children and Youth.* Elk Grove Village, IL, American Academy of Pediatrics (in press)
3. *A Handbook for Public Playground Safety,* Vol. I. General guidelines for new and existing playgrounds. Washington, DC: US Consumer Product Safety Commission, 1981, p 3
4. Occupational Safety and Health Administration, General Industry Standard, 29-CFR 1910.23 C1.
5. *A Handbook for Public Playground Safety,* Vol. II. Technical guidelines for equipment and surfacing. Washington, DC: US Consumer Product Safety Commission, 1981, p 15
6. Consumer Product Safety Commission, 16 CFR Chapter II, *Federal Register,* 1979;44:57353
7. *Code for Safety to Life from Fire in Buildings and Structures.* Quincy, MA, National Fire Protection Association, 1985
8. *A Design Guide for Home Safety.* US Department of Housing and Urban Development. Washington, DC: US Government Printing Office, 1972, pp 2-9 (out of print)
9. National Highway Transportation Safety Administration: *19 City Survey.* March 1985
10. Ziegler P: Child safety seat misuse. *Research Notes,* National Highway Transportation Safety Administration, January 1985

Chapter 7

HEALTH TRAINING FOR CHILD CARE STAFF

7.1 Who Works In Child Care

Instructors who plan training curricula for caregivers should be aware of the diversity of individuals who work in child care programs. Child care staff persons originate from two sources: some are graduates of two- or four-year colleges and Master's degree programs; others are paraprofessionals who have ascended the child care career ladder through inservice training.[1,2] Undergraduate courses designed to prepare college students for child care work are found in departments of early childhood education, home economics (or human ecology), psychology, and social work. Paraprofessionals participate in on-the-job training at community colleges, in courses supervised by a national credentialing system called the Child Development Associate Consortium,[3] in training programs arranged by employers or funding agencies, and in individually designed activities at the child care center where the staff member is employed.

Women constitute the majority of child caregivers, although the number of men in the field is slowly increasing.[4,5] Most have some education beyond high school and almost all are grossly underpaid by any standard. Despite their education, training, and responsibility, child care workers are among the lowest wage earners in the country with few, if any, fringe benefits.[6] Salaries, which are frequently below the poverty level, contribute to a high turnover of staff members and a decrease in the quality of care. It is not unusual to have half the staff turn over every two years. Because new personnel are constantly being oriented and trained, education of the staff in child care programs must be continuous.

7.2 Wants versus Needs for Training

At present, in most child care training curricula there is little, if any, teaching of health, safety, and nutrition. Although training for work with children consistently emphasizes the "whole child," these topics are largely ignored; there is no textbook or specific set of materials that treats health, safety, and nutrition in day care adequately, and few curricula have established courses to prepare the student to deal with them. Instructors who want to incorporate child health issues into their training presentation must gather materials, extract relevant information, and synthesize readings for the students. The unmet need for information on these subjects can be filled by pediatricians who participate in day care training courses given at selected day care sites, at a sponsoring agency community room, and at a local community college classroom.

Workers in child care need to know how to promote health and safety in the child care setting—and how to do it with few financial resources and usually with no health professionals on the site. Child care staff members have to know how to deal with common health problems (from chicken pox to bruises), how to obtain health professional services when they are needed, and how to maintain standards of health and safety which protect children from injury and illness. Job-related stress and the absence of tangible rewards for good performance are challenging obstacles to the development of the expertise required of adults who have so much responsibility for care of young children.

Often, child care workers want to focus on training in the areas that cause them anxiety, even though they may need training in other areas as well. Adults who come to work in child care are generally eager to learn, although they usually bring with them the mixture of old wives' tales and health beliefs they learned in their own childhood and from their life experience. They recognize that because parents look to them as child care experts, they must learn as much as they can to do their job well. Caregivers want information about recognition and management of infectious diseases; they also need to know about measures which will help prevent such diseases from occurring in the first place. Caregivers show great interest in learning first aid, but they also need to learn how to recognize and reduce hazards which cause injuries.

Many caregivers are fascinated by medical techniques. For example, it is not uncommon for caregivers to want to learn cardiopulmonary resuscitation although they do not know how to handle lacerations properly. Child care staff members believe that they need a medical authority to specify the criteria used to determine when sick children should be excluded from and readmitted to day care; they want to know what commercial product kills germs and how to use it on toys and surfaces; how to get information from doctors that is helpful in planning care for the child; how caregivers can stay well. These issues are important. Some of them can be addressed by a member of the child care staff who has been trained by a medical expert; others should be explained by a health professional directly. Once the facts and the rationale governing good health practice have been made clear, the child care staff and the parents of children in the program must evolve the policies appropriate to the specific child care setting.

The designer of a training program has to keep in mind the distinction between the training that is wanted and the training that is needed. To capture the interest of caregivers, some of what is wanted must be addressed, but what is needed must also be included. The program should be aimed at areas of concern to the trainees, whether the training is for students who are not yet employed or for child care workers on the job. The scheduling of sessions is also important. Courses for employed caregivers in a college setting are best given in the evenings or on weekends. If the training is to take place during child care hours, the two-hour nap period in the early afternoon is usually used when substitute caregivers can supervise sleeping children. Some administrators set aside certain days annually in which the care program is closed for staff workshops and inservice training. Because of the burden that lack of day care services places on working parents, the nap-time, evening, or weekend times are most commonly used. Use of these periods represents an infringement on caregivers' precious personal recovery time. The contribution of the participants in relinquishing their time deserves recognition, and thoughtful planning is obligatory to minimize the stress they incur.

7.3 Topics to Cover in Training

Although some staff members, especially in large day care centers, may be hired for specific duties and instructed in their performance only, it is usually desirable to design a training program that surveys the broad range of topics fundamental to expert day care service. The health professional who is called upon to contribute to the training program should be sure that the following health and safety topics are included:

Child health:	Relationship to learning ability
	Relationship to health in adulthood
Health assessment:	Description of routine methods
	What is usually found
	Scheduling health assessments
	Function of routine health care in tracking development and preventing illness
	Screening to find specific health problems
	Early detection as an aid to prevention and treatment
	Evaluation of hearing, speech, vision, and dental problems
Health records:	Information to collect
	How to store it and how to use it
	Problems of access; confidentiality
	Transfer and disposal of records
Access to health care services:	How to get health care in the community

Where day care administrators can find advice and service

Using health consultants

Working with health professionals as part of the child's health care team

Obtaining care: parental versus staff members' responsibility

Mental health services:

When are they required?

Observation to assess behavior and development

How to locate and use mental health services

Health policies:

Evaluation of the health component of child care

Setting and communicating standards for healthy behaviors

Health education for children and parents

Resources and personnel for health education

Written health policies and procedures for all health-related aspects of the program

Nutrition:

Good nutrition for children at different developmental stages

How to implement good nutrition in day care for infants, toddlers, preschoolers, and school-aged children

Food preparation; snack and meal service

Nutrition problems

Illness:

Recognizing symptoms of acute illness

Managing the sick child

Administering medication

When to call a health professional

Caring for children with chronic illnesses

Infection: Infectious diseases to which children are susceptible

Why ear infections are common in children

How infectious diseases are transmitted

Child care as a factor in the risk of infection

How to prevent and manage infectious diseases in the child care setting (immunizations, sanitation)

Practical procedures to solve problems in containing infection

When and who to call to report an infectious disease problem

Sources of information about infectious disease for program staff.

Safety: Prevention of injury through hazard detection and elimination

Promoting safety without limiting joy or making a lot of extra work

Recording and reporting injuries

First aid

Emergency preparedness; emergency contact and consent forms

Arrangement for contacting parents in emergencies

Disaster plans

	Minimizing risks: seeking help from community resources
Children with disabilities:	How to care for them
	How health professionals help
	Special needs of parents of children with disabilities
Abused and neglected children:	Recognizing abuse and neglect
	Reporting cases of abuse and neglect
	Finding help and handling feelings
	Dealing with families under stress

Some materials and sources useful in developing training for child care workers are listed in Appendix VI.1.

7.4 Methods of Training

Methods of training vary from informal instruction by visiting experts to planned classroom sessions. One of the least expensive forms of staff training is the exchange that takes place between state licensing personnel and caregivers during the on-site visits that are a part of the licensing process. Under the watchful eye of an inspector, caregivers think about correct procedures and try to conform to the requirements being used to measure their performance. Veteran licensing inspectors and the monitors sent by state and municipal agencies offer comments and suggestions that are regarded by caregivers as helpful. In general, child care staff members are eager to do the right thing when they know what the right thing is.

The approach used in formal coursework is as important as the content. The first step in planning a successful program is to assess the needs and wants of the group to be addressed. Needs may be determined by data gathered from the students at the beginning of a course, or, for staff members of a particular child care program, by a review of licensing data or by an evaluation of current practices in use at the care center. Information can be gathered by using questionnaires and on-site observation routines that have been developed to assess the adequacy of the health component of child care programs.[7] In many states observers use checklists based on the requirements of licensing regulations. However, these checklists are not an adequate test of what caregivers need to know because the licensing regulations represent only minimum compliance with protective requirements, not the full range of desirable practices. Further exploration is necessary. A questionnaire should outline the general issues relevant to children's health care and ask potential trainees to rank their priorities among the topics. The questionnaire should also provide an opportunity to suggest additional topics of concern. Group discussions should focus on problems and areas of uncertainty that the trainees want to discuss.

Using data gathered from the assessment, the instructor can refine the training plan. Although it may be tedious to write out a detailed plan for each session, the quality of the training will be much improved by the discipline of such preparation. Lesson plans should include objectives, concepts to be covered, methods to be used, materials and equipment required, the timing for each activity, and a plan for the evaluation of each activity. Evaluation plans should be tied to behavioral objectives wherever possible. (See Appendix VII.1 for a training plan form.)

On-the-job training is enhanced when trainees have an opportunity to teach the techniques that they have just learned. Supervisors can be asked to provide a scheduled opportunity for the student to "teach back" the material covered in a session to coworkers who did not attend. Teaching peers reinforces learning and provides an opportunity for discussions that result in practical suggestions for change.

An effective technique for starting training sessions is to ask the participants to introduce themselves and state their expectations of the training experience. This "warm-up" time pays rich dividends by revealing to the instructor the hidden agendas and priorities of students. Using name tags with first names for everyone, including the instructor, is usually welcomed by child care personnel. It is particularly helpful when a physician is willing to be called by her or his first name. The warm-up activity should be followed by a review of the agenda for the training period so that students are clear about what is planned for them.

Teaching methods that are most likely to produce behavioral changes are those that involve the student in some active way. For example, during discussions of playground safety, trainees can be asked to evaluate and suggest affordable safety modifications for their own playground or for a neighborhood, using information on hazards and safe playground design provided by the instructor. A demonstration of correct hand washing technique is an effective training method, especially when it is followed by student hand washing before refreshments are served. There are topics, however, that do not lend themselves easily to hands-on learning techniques. To cover these, instructors often resort to the lecture method. Although lectures are an efficient way to communicate facts, they are the least effective way to accomplish behavioral change. It is better to develop the material through group discussions which draw on personal experiences of the trainees. Audiovisual aids (films, slides, handouts, demonstrations) should be liberally used, but they should be varied and not prolonged. (See Appendix VII.2 for Medical Terms handout.) Pacing of the training to limit passive activities to no more than 30 minutes at a time is a good idea.

7.5 Physical Environment for Training

The setting in which the training is conducted is important to the outcome. The students' attention and involvement are enhanced by having seats arranged in a semicircle with as few additional rows of chairs as possible. Where available, tables help to keep handouts in view and provide a surface to lean on. A horseshoe-shaped arrangement of tables is most desirable. The ideal group size is between ten and 20 trainees. Fewer than ten may produce too little input for lively discussions. More than 20 makes individual participation difficult. Except when the group is so large that there is no alternative, classroom-style seating in rows should be avoided. Good lighting, comfortable chairs, and comfortable room temperature also help in effective training.

7.6 Health Professionals as Trainers

Many health professionals can be health trainers for child care personnel, but some will be better than others. It takes a certain amount of showmanship to be an effective teacher. Additionally, it helps if there is an opportunity for repeated contact between the trainer and the students. Learning then becomes continuous; students can keep up with changing knowledge and deepen their understanding of health and safety issues. Because local providers of health care are more likely to be available for continuing contact, they are a potential source of good trainers.

Few day care programs can afford to pay much if anything for the training their staff members need. Many programs depend upon health department nurses or pediatricians who care for some of the children in the program as sources of donated or low-cost training. However, day care personnel pay richly in gratitude for any health professional input. Whether practitioners are paid or contribute their time to provide training to child care staff, their reward comes from the knowledge that many children are likely to benefit from the information they impart.

References

1. Ruopp R, Travers J, Glantz F, et al: *Children at the Center.* Cambridge, MA, Abt Books, 1979, p 213
2. Devine-Hawkins P: *Family Day Care in the United States.* DHHS Pub. No. (OHDS) 80-30287. Washington, DC: US Government Printing Office, 1981, pp 13-14
3. Child Development Associates National Credentialing Program. 1341 G Street NW, Suite 802, Washington, DC 20005. 1-800-424-4310
4. Ruopp R, et al: *Children at the Center,* p 212, table 15
5. Devine-Hawkins P: *Family Day Care in the United States,* p 11
6. Morgan G: Child care options for working parents, in Sharp, M (ed): *Daycare.* Report of the Sixteenth Ross Roundtable. Columbus, OH, Ross Laboratories, 1985, p 7
7. Aronson SS, Aiken LS: Compliance of child care programs with health and safety standards: Impact of program evaluation and advocate training. PEDIATRICS 1980;65:318-325

Bibliography

Mager RF: *Preparing Instructional Objectives*. Palo Alto, CA, Fearon Publishers, Inc, 1962

Mager, RF: *Developing Attitude Toward Learning*. Belmont, CA, Lear Siegler, Inc/Fearon Publishers, 1968

Mager, RF: *Measuring Instructional Intent (or got a match?)* Belmont, CA, Lear Siegler, Inc/Fearon Publishers, 1973

Mager, RF, Beach KM, Jr: *Developing Vocational Instruction*. Belmont, CA, Lear Siegler, Inc/Fearon Publishers, 1967

Chapter 8

THE HEALTH PROFESSIONAL AS A HEALTH CONSULTANT TO DAY CARE PROGRAMS

8.1 Introduction

Health professionals may play many roles in community child care and day care. In practice, as child or family health consultants, they may counsel parents about educational and child care arrangements and about behavior and management of children in the home and out of it. They may resolve problems directly or recommend specific resources from which help can be sought. They may teach child development, child care, and child rearing. Health professionals may also work or lobby for improved child care and day care facilities nationally or in their local communities. In addition, they may be asked to act as consultants to family day care providers, center staff, or agencies. Some of these roles may be unfamiliar ones for health professionals trained to work with individual patients and families.

8.2 Counseling Roles

Health professionals may be asked for advice or information on a particular issue, for help with an individual child, or for broad guidance in making a day care center an optimal environment for the healthy development of children. In a program already in operation, the health professional may find himself or herself the sole source of advice or one of a number of consultants providing help. The consultant may be asked to speak with caregivers about the physical or mental health of a child or to talk with the child's parents. There may be a need for group discussions with parents or staff members about issues of general interest. Administrators might want the health professional's assistance in revamping health maintenance procedures, implementing a plan already in hand, or training staff members responsible for executing one. A health professional whose child is in the program may be asked to involve himself or herself actively as a parent.

Health professionals are also called upon as consultants when a care program is in the planning stage. In this case, there is an opportunity to institute good health practices from the beginning and often to see that the physical facilities are modified to support them. The health professional may be the best person to plead the case of the day care center before community agencies whose cooperation is needed.

8.3 The Health Component and the Health Consultant

Almost everything that goes on in a day care center and almost everything about the center itself affects the health of the children it serves. The health consultant has to define the aspects of care, activity, physical maintenance, and administration that relate to the prevention of illness and injury, the management of both, and the enhancement of the child's development, treating these as the "health component" of the program that is his or her province.

Each health professional will subdivide the health component differently, but every consultant's list should cover:
1. Health services—screening, medical evaluation, and treatment
2. Special services for children with disabilities or chronic illnesses and for abused or neglected children
3. Dental hygiene
4. Health records for children, staff, and volunteers
5. Health and mental health education for staff, parents, and children
6. Staff health and mental health
7. First aid
8. Evacuation, emergency, and disaster plans
9. Environmental quality and safety, including transportation and playground safety
10. Nutrition
11. Health policies and procedures
12. Linkage with community resources for health care

Few, if any, health professionals are experts in all the areas that comprise the health component of child care. As a rule, a practitioner who is consulted should give advice about the things that he or she is qualified by training and experience to judge, calling on other community professionals for counsel when the need arises. (See Appendix VI.1 for a list of typical community resources to which health consultants can go for information, and Appendix VIII for additional reading on the general aspects of day care.)

8.4 Acting as a Health Consultant: Preliminary Steps

The first step in the consultative process should be the matching of the priorities of the consultant and the personnel at the child care facility. An effective consultant listens carefully to what is said about the needs of the program but also looks for themes underlying the consultation request. Is there some problem that is not being verbalized and is there a "hidden agenda"? An understanding of the philosophy of the program, its staff, and the roles and relationships of its personnel is essential for successful consultation. The planning and implementation of good health and safety practices requires close cooperation and mutual understanding between the director and staff of the child care facility and the health consultant. In addition, the consultant should be cognizant of the lifestyles of the families served, the parent-child relationships within these families, and the relationships between the families and the personnel at the care center.

The consultant should determine, at the outset, what the directors of the care center hope to achieve. Unrealistic expectations can doom a consultation to failure. Are the issues or problems specific or is the consultation meant to effect general improvement? The health professional should find out who will be the "contact person" from the center with whom he or she will work, whether this individual is responsible for the health component of the program, and whether any other health specialists are already involved. If the consultant's services are to be paid, the financial arrangements should be settled. Finally, the health professional and the contact person should work out a mutually satisfactory plan of action, determine the form in which the consultant will convey recommendations, and decide who will be responsible for acting upon them.

In initial meetings with the director or the staff member who is the contact person, the consultant gathers background information about the program by asking questions about the services, the staff, and the parents and children involved. Brochures or handouts distributed by the center should be read and a review made of the existing health policies and programs. The consultant ought to explore the relationship between the care center and the community at large.

Having ascertained the nature of the care facility, the health professional ought then to investigate the health care resources available to it in the community. Is there assistance that can be rendered by private physicians or other health practitioners, or by public clinics, health departments, community health and mental health centers, or dental programs? What about the efforts of service clubs and other public and voluntary groups? In making his or her recommendations, the consultant should be aware of community services already in place and avoid suggesting duplication. He or she ought also to become familiar with state and local licensing requirements, especially in the areas of health, nutrition or feeding programs, sanitation, safety, and caregiving personnel. Requirements, in written form, are available from state or county departments of health, social service, or education.

At this point, the consultant is prepared to meet with individuals and groups associated with the day care center to extend his or her investigation. In conversing with administrators, directors or trustees, staff persons, or parents or representatives of the Parents' Group (if there is one), the consultant should listen to their view of the facility's philosophy, policies, and procedures, always sensitive to the attitudes and aims of the speakers. Evaluating their contribution to the program and their skills, the consultant should find out how they feel about the health issues, what they think they need, and what they would like to have done. Search for any relationships, existing or potential, that individuals may have with members of the medical community like public health nurses, nurse practitioners, or primary care physicians. Is there a parent who is a health professional?

8.5 Planning and Implementation of a Health Program

The success of any health program encompassing preventive principles is contingent on the cooperation of the administration and the staff of the child care program. For this reason every effort should be made to plan inexpensive and easily implemented procedures. *One person in the program must be designated as the individual responsible for the health program.* Although this person may have other responsibilities in addition to the supervision of the health component, and others may help implement health activities, accountability for health matters must be clearly assigned to one staff member.

Definable health goals, a method for evaluating health policy in relation to the goals, and methods for implementing necessary changes are essential. Child care programs provide an opportunity for assuring optimal health care for participating children and their families. Improving health care begins with the identification of existing problems, and screening procedures can be used as a first step in this process. The problems that screening doesn't catch are likely to appear to caregivers or parents observing the children in their activities. With this in mind, the consultant helping in the development of a health program should recommend the following:

1. Someone on the staff of the child care program should assume responsibility for the health program.
2. Health screening and management plans should be tailored, not only to each child, but to the children as a group with attention paid to socio-economic status and ethnocultural patterns. Any plan should either bring services to the children or the children to the services in a way fitting parents' working hours, finances, and ability to cope with the local health care system.
3. A plan for the training and involvement of staff members should be developed to assure their access to pertinent health information.
4. Parents should be involved in all decisions relating to the health of the children, whether in the area of program planning or problem-solving.
5. Staff members should periodically review the health program.

For medical services for the children who do not have their own physician, a liaison with a private or public clinic or health service group that has an on-going screening and preventive program may be worthwhile. This liaison may provide basic care for children unable to secure private care. For all children, screening procedures are not always available in private offices, e.g., audiometry, assessment of visual acuity, anemia screening and specific developmental testing. The consultant is in an excellent position to recommend screening resources in the community as well as resources for follow-up and remediation if the families are unable to find appropriate resources on their own. The consultant's knowledge of the health care system and community resources will be of great value to child care administrators and staff members unfamiliar with the health scene.

8.6 Illness, Emergencies, and Safety

The health consultant will become involved in the controversial issue of the handling of the child who is brought to day care with a minor illness or becomes ill during the day. Policies and procedures will vary from facility to facility and community to community, depending on many factors including the physical facilities, staff attitudes, and capabilities. The support available from the medical community makes a difference in what can be done and so does the attitude, resources, and availability of the parents. A number of day care centers have developed creative plans for coping with this problem, such as a cadre of parents or grandparents who agree to volunteer as babysitters for the sick child in the child's own home. Finding alternate sources of child care for children excluded for longer term health reasons is another problem faced by many consultants. (See Programs for Sick Child Care in Chapter V, Section 5.7.C.)

The health consultant should assist the child care staff in

1. Identifying at least one member of the staff who is either knowledgeable, or willing to be extensively trained in first aid procedures. This could be the person who is responsible for the total health program or another member of the staff. All child care personnel should acquire a rudimen-

tary knowledge of first aid and the treatment of minor injuries.

2. Developing a written policy and standing orders for handling minor injuries, illnesses, and special health problems. Written policies relating to emergencies should deal with issues such as parental permission for emergency care, consent forms, transportation, and available physicians, clinics, and hospitals.

3. Planning for medical or nursing backup for child care personnel when problems arise. A community physician, clinic, or nurse should be available for telephone consultation at all times. In some communities, several centers join in funding one nurse or nurse practitioner.

4. Establishing criteria for the exclusion of sick children and considering alternate child care options for children of working parents if exclusion is deemed necessary. Parents should be informed of these criteria prior to the enrollment of their child in the center or program.

5. Developing policies and procedures for the admission and care of such ill children if it is legal in a particular state. Include the allocation of appropriate space to assure the sick child comfort and privacy under supervision of an adequate number of trained staff members (including caregivers whom the child knows), the establishment of standing orders relative to medications, and the development of guidelines concerning parent and/or volunteer involvement.

6. Developing criteria for the acceptance of children with disabilities into the day care program and guidelines for their special care.

7. Defining the roles of parents, staff, and administrators in planning and implementing health and safety policies and procedures.

8. Establishing basic sanitation and safety standards for providing a safe and healthy environment (higher than minimum licensing requirements) and arranging for evaluation and reevaluation to be sure these standards are met.

8.7 Health Policies and Instruction for Staff Members

Staff members of a day care center assure the health of the children in two ways: they maintain their own health by good practices that serve as models for the children to copy, and they adhere to procedures that limit the spread of infection and promote safety. The health consultant should assist administrators in spelling out the policies and training agenda that make staff members effective health promoters.

A statement should be developed covering the standard of personal health required of caregivers. It should specify the health screening to be used, schedule for physical examinations, and criteria for exclusion or mandatory remediation. There may be special arrangements for health consultation, and the policies for sick leave and maternity leave should be determined.

The health professional can describe the subject matter that ought to be conveyed to the staff in training sessions (see chapter VII). Caregivers must have a clear idea of what to watch for as signs of health and illness and clues to abuse or neglect. Instruction should make them confident about responding to injury, sudden illness, chronic health problems, and disabilities. They should know when to call for outside help. A well-planned training course embracing this material can prepare staff members to act as auxiliary health educators for the children and their parents.

8.8 Advising Staff Members Caring for Very Young Children

In addition to assisting the child care staff in programs offering care for older children, the health consultant to facilities providing child care to infants and toddlers should assist the child care staff in

1. Developing written policies and procedures for infant safety, the care of diapers and designation of separate diaper change areas, type and method of feeding, clothing changes, hand washing, type of bed or crib, care of linen, and the cleaning of chairs, tables, toys, utensils, and cribs.
2. Establishing a plan for daily health appraisal of the infants by the staff.
3. Arranging for frequent or constant on-site health guidance from a registered nurse or perhaps a licensed practical nurse on the child care staff or by special arrangement with a visiting nurse or with a health facility.

8.9 Mental Health Consultation

Many health professionals do not feel prepared to serve as mental health consultants and would be more comfortable calling in someone with special mental health expertise when this kind of advice is needed. The following are potential sources of mental health support for the consultant and for the program:
1. Private community resources
   a. Pediatricians, family physicians, and nurse practitioners with special interest and training in child development and family counseling
   b. Child psychiatrists and child psychologists
   c. Social workers and family counselors
2. Mental health services, child guidance clinics and family service agencies
3. Child psychiatry and pediatric divisions of medical centers and children's hospitals
4. Religious organizations and community service clubs
5. Public school departments
6. Colleges and universities
   a. Early childhood education and child development programs
   b. Psychology, education, guidance and counseling, and social work departments

8.10 Health Education

A child care setting offers almost limitless opportunities for health education. After consulting with the staff and the administration, a health professional can make specific recommendations for health education curricula for children, staff, and parents. Topics to include are child development, parent-child relationships, behavior management and discipline, nutrition, dental health, physical fitness, safety, special needs of the child with disabilities, and disease prevention. The consultant can make specific recommendations to the director or to whomever is designated as the health person or health advocate within the facility or program. By calling upon community agencies for guest speakers, handouts, and ideas for activities, the person in charge can design a rich and creative program.

8.11 Summary

The health consultant to a child care program should talk with everyone involved with the facility but must have a link to the administrative authority so that his or her recommendations can be implemented. This should be made clear at the beginning so that the consultant's efforts will bear fruit. In this kind of consultation, the ability to listen and offer advice on the topics the health consultant deems important as well as those the care providers specify will determine success or failure.

The consultant who prepares himself or herself for the task will also be most effective. A good consultant, whether coming in for a single visit or several, will read any written material supplied by the care center and will give some thought to the community it serves, to state and county licensing requirements, and to the health resources available in the community.

The effective consultant will also ask to meet with staff members and representative parents rather than just an administrator or the director. Policy setting and decision-making in concert with staff members and parents have the best chance of success. In addition, parent involvement minimizes the possibility of insensitivity, or even worse, abuse on the part of the program administrators and staff members.

Throughout this chapter the importance of one staff member serving as health coordinator or health advocate has been emphasized. Care centers that can afford a part-time or full-time health professional to take this responsibility have the best opportunity to develop a strong health component.

In the past, health professionals have not been trained to serve as consultants to other than medical programs. Aware of the growing number of children whose health is affected by day care, many physicians in charge of pediatric training programs are incorporating experiences that will prepare practitioners to advise caregivers. In some parts of the country, local pediatric committees and task forces are beginning to work with child care and early childhood education organizations such as the National Association for the Education of Young Children and its local affiliates to provide the kind of health care that each child needs and all children should enjoy.

References

1. Aronson SS: Health Consultation in Child Care. *Day Care and Early Education*, Fall, 1983, pp 26-32
2. Aronson SS: Health consultation in day care, in Auerbach S (ed): *Model Programs and Their Components.* New York, Human Sciences Press, 1976
3. BANANAS, Child Care Information and Referral and Parent Support, 6501 Telegraph Ave., Oakland, CA 94609, 1980
4. Clarke SA: *Day Care.* Cambridge, MA, Harvard University Press, 1982
5. Friedman D, Sale J, Weinstein V: *Child Care and the Family.* Chicago, National Committee for the Prevention of Child Abuse, 1985
6. Healy A, Friedman D: The health professional and day care for young children, in Wallace H, et al (ed): *Maternal and Child Health Practices*, ed 2. New York, John Wiley and Sons, 1982

7. Heinicke C, Sale J, Prescott E, Puncel C, Friedman D: Organization of day care: Considerations relating to the mental health of child and family. *Am J Orthopsychiatry* 1973;43:8-22
8. Kiester DJ: *Consultation in Day Care.* Chapel Hill, NC, University of North Carolina, 1969
9. Zigler E, Gordon E (eds): *Day Care: Scientific and Social Policy Issues.* Boston, Auburn House, 1982

Chapter 9

DAY CARE REGULATIONS, HEALTH POLICIES AND THEIR ADMINISTRATION

9.1 Introduction

All pediatricians volunteering to serve on a local health advisory council or preparing to provide consultation to a child care facility, to advise a family regarding the use of day care, or to represent a medical association in advocating day care legislation, regulations, and licensing should understand the organization of the day care system nationally and in their own state. They should recognize how they can contribute to raising the standards for child care through the role they are about to play.

9.2 Status of Day Care Regulations

At the present time there are no federal regulations directed specifically to the general health of children in day care. Although federal regulations have been developed, they were suspended in 1980. The decision to hold back is related in part to the value placed by the federal government on family privacy and parents' responsibility for child rearing. The federal government does, however, heavily subsidize day care for low-income families and provide tax credits for middle- and upper-income working parents who use day care. Project Head Start is a federally subsidized comprehensive developmental service for preschool children from low-income families which has developed and continues to provide program performance standards for each child's growth and development. These performance standards are available to any group providing preschool child care programs.[1]

Licensing is the responsibility of state government. Licensing reduces the chance of harm to children in out-of-home care. Legal enforcement is a mechanism for correcting deficiencies. The choice of agency to develop licensing standards varies from state to state. In many states, the responsibility is assigned to the state's social service agency or a special office for children. In other states, it rests with the Department of Health. There is great need to increase the specificity of day care regulations that pertain to the promotion of the health of children and staff members and to the prevention and management of injury and illness. The minimal regulations currently in effect in many states allow varied interpretations and great likelihood of poor health practices. These may result in dysfunctional social behaviors in the child, frequent minor and occasional severe injuries, presence of preventable illness, and spread of contagious diseases.[2]

Every state requires licensing of day care. Some states do not regulate or license family day care, and some exempt care that is church-sponsored. Regulations have been developed primarily to protect children from physical and psychological insults. In personal health, they govern mandated health examinations for children and staff, immunizations, nutrition, and exclusion of children from care. In environmental health, the regulations relate to sanitation, emergency procedures, and safety.[3] Although they continue to be revised and improved, regulations are still less precise than some health professionals would like and are still sometimes illogical, inappropriate for unique programs, and costly to meet. Aware of these imperfections, knowledgeable professionals work for changes and emphasize that regulations should be reviewed at least every five years to respond to new knowledge.

The most pressing need is for regulations that apply to the care of very young children because the demand for day care for the infant and toddler is now growing rapidly. Currently, there are very limited regulations in most states for this group of children. Because of the infant's particular sensitivity to environmental input, licensing standards and policies for this group require constructive thought and action at this time.[4]

Federal legislation regarding components of child care is generally intended for the improvement of care. How it is implemented in the states may affect day care subsidies, e.g., Title XX. With new federal legislation, new state statutes must be developed, old ones may have to be amended, and new regulations must be written; training for licensing personnel and education of child care providers and parents about new rulings must be provided in some fashion.[5] The nationwide activity following the recent passage of legislation responding to cases of child abuse in child care settings (Public Law 98-473) is a good example of this process.[6]

9.3 The Role of Licensing Personnel

Licensing agency staff members have traditionally interpreted day care requirements and helped day care operators to comply. It is important to know the qualifications of licensing personnel in one's own state and to what extent they are able to provide training and technical assistance as well as perform their licensing function. Usually these staff persons need training in the same areas as the child care providers. It is also important to know in one's own state how often licensing personnel are able to visit care facilities and whether they inspect day care programs that are required to be registered but not licensed. (In some places the latter may not be visited at all.) Reduction in funds may increase the volume of work required of a licensing worker, decrease qualifications required for the job, limit the number of visits, and reduce the opportunity to provide training and technical assistance to child care providers.[7] In many states local health department sanitarians may apply health codes developed for other institutions to day care settings. Such conflicting requirements should be avoided. In some states a visit by a health professional to day care programs is not routine. In these states, an inspector may go to a day care facility only when a complaint is received.

9.4 Health Care Policies

Health care policies are a recorded documentation of a definite method of action developed by a single center, a group of centers, or even a designated community group. The policies should be designed to protect and promote the health of the children in care. Topics to be covered are essentially those listed in Chapter VII, Section 7.3.

Every child care facility should adopt a health policy. State standards, rules, regulations, and recommendations may be used as a base. In some communities day care health policies are not only more specific than state licensing requirements, but demand the institution and maintenance of a higher quality of care. These policies usually reflect the community's understanding of the importance of a health component in day care and sometimes reflect the attitude of a health advisory committee.

The health advisory committee may be a standing committee of a child care agency board, an *ad hoc* committee, or a community health council supervising a number of day care programs. Its membership should include parents who use day care, practicing physicians, public health nurses, building inspectors, representatives from the local health department, fire marshall's office, the consumer safety association, and others who are knowledgeable and interested. A standing committee is preferable to an *ad hoc* committee as policies require periodic reviews and revisions. Its leadership is critical and requires a person committed to the importance of day care of good quality.

A staff person with training in child or public health should be designated by each program, whether small or large, to implement the health policies that have been accepted by the governing body of the child care program. This person should have access to local and state health consultants as well as the health advisory committee. The staff person should be directly responsible to the chief administrator of the program. In a small program, the program director might be the staff person responsible for the administration of health policy.

Individual physicians and state medical society representatives should be advocates for day care legislation that provides specific regulations supportive of the health of children. Physicians are also strongly urged to offer guidance for the development of these regulations, to participate in the establishment of health policies, and to assist in the training of the personnel who implement them.

References

1. Head Start Bureau, Administration for Children, Youth and Families, Office of Human Development Services, US Department of Health and Human Services, Washington, DC 20013.
2. Morgan G: Regulatory gaps and excesses. Symposium on infectious diseases in day care: Management and prevention. Minneapolis, MN, June 1984 (in press)
3. Schloesser PT, Cameron EE, Class N, Norris S: Kansas public health intervention to reduce risks for children in day care. Paper presented at American Public Health Association. San Francisco, November 1984 (unpublished)
4. Young K, Zigler E: Infant and toddler day care: Regulations and
   . policy implications. *Am J Orthopsychiatry* 1986;56:43-55
5. Blank H, Comstock-Gay L: Issues to consider in developing legislation concerning background checks for child care providers as well as other equally important initiatives to help to improve families' access to quality child care. Washington, DC: Children's Defense Fund, 1985. (Direct request for paper to the authors, c/o The Children's Defense Fund, 122 C Street NW, Washington, DC 20001.)
6. Cohen AJ: Vigilant in the protection of our children or vigilantes? Legal considerations in drafting screening laws and recommendations for safeguarding children in child care settings. San Francisco: Child Care Law Center, 1985. (Direct request for paper to Abby J. Cohen, Managing Attorney, Child Care Law Center, 625 Market St. #815, San Francisco, CA 94105.)
7. Kendall ED, Walker L: Day care licensing: The eroding regulations. *Child Care Quarterly* 1984;13:278-290
8. Aronson SS: Health update: Health policies and procedures. *Child Care Information Exchange*, September/October 1983

APPENDIX I.1

THE PEDIATRICIAN'S ROLE IN PROMOTING THE HEALTH OF A PATIENT IN DAY CARE*

American families have changed. More mothers are working, and more young children are being cared for outside the home. The stresses inherent in this sociologic change are great.

Pediatric practice has also changed. Increasingly, pediatricians are involved not only in the medical care of the child, but in the ecologic system in which the child exists. The pediatrician has traditionally worked with parents and children to promote healthy functioning, which encompasses the physical, emotional, cognitive, and social health of the growing and developing child. Now, the pediatrician must expand this role to include working with significant other adults who interact closely with the child who spends much of the day away from home. In this way, the pediatrician will contribute to the promotion of the child's general well-being, and some maladaptive behaviors will be prevented.

Parents and adults whom parents delegate to provide child care on a regular basis have the greatest responsibility for children. With increasing numbers of single-parent families and families in which both parents work, there is a greater use of the variety of alternative caregiving arrangements involving adults who are neither parents nor relatives of the child. Effective communication among the child's pediatrician and regular caregivers is more difficult to achieve than in the past when parents provided most of the child's care. When developmental irregularities or a chronic illness are a concern, it is particularly important for pediatricians to communicate to the person(s) providing child care the unique features of the child and family. Thus the caregiver will be

*This statement has been approved by the Council on Child and Adolescent Health.
PEDIATRICS (ISSN 0031 4005). Copyright 1984 by the American Academy of Pediatrics.
PEDIATRICS Vol. 74 No.1 July 1984

better able to prepare an individualized program that enhances the child's development, increases self-esteem, and supports the parents' child-caring capacity.

Current methods of communication between pediatricians and child care providers are often woefully inadequate. Much useful and important data are not shared. Often, the child care provider receives only certification of immunization status and documentation of a visit to the pediatrician's office. In providing continuing health care for the child, the pediatrician acquires a great deal of information about the child's medical status, adaptability, and temperament, as well as family strengths. This information could be used to enhance the family's successful use of a day care resource. Pediatricians underestimate the value of this wealth of information they have gathered, and it is often only loosely documented in the child's health profile required for entry into a day care setting. Conversely, pediatricians could increase their understanding of the child and contribute more effectively to the child's growth and development with access to the behavioral observations made by the significant adults involved in the child's day care program.

In order to advise the family about whether day care is timely, or to counsel the family regarding preparation for the separation, or to answer such questions as, "Is this a good setting for my child?" and "Is the child able to participate in all aspects of the day care program?," the pediatrician must not only know the child and the family, but must have some understanding of the specific programs. Will the day care program be supportive to the family's parenting style? Will the parent be able to participate in decisions regarding the child's daily activities? Can the staff adapt to the parents' needs? Can the staff members show spontaneous affection? Is there a schedule of activities? Is nutritious food provided? What accident precautions are enforced on special trips? What are the sanitary precautions for the care of the young child? What are the policies regarding the ill child? Is there an identified staff person responsible for issues related to health? Is the program licensed? Most of these questions may be answered by a parent; others may be answered by the program director or the local licensing agency. Most, but not all, needs can be met.

In the child's best interest, there should be a system for exchanging information about the child between the physician and the day care provider. This exchange is generally infrequent and used primarily to understand a child for whom there is concern, e.g., the child with asthma, the clumsy child, or the child who is less or more mature than his or her chronologic age expectations. The parent will usually be transmitting his or her own concerns and the concerns raised by the two systems, but with prior approval from the parent, telephone calls and/or notes between physician and day care provider may be more efficient and effective.

Common topics for communication between a physician and a day care provider may include: (1) current state of health and nutrition, including management of colds, diarrhea, bruises, chronic illness, handicapping conditions, and poor or exuberant appetite; (2) growth pattern observed over time and its significance to physical adaptation in the day care environment, such as size of chairs, height of steps, fatigue; (3) hearing and vision function, e.g., the child with recurrent middle ear effusion who may be irritable and unresponsive to auditory stimuli or the child who requires glasses but doesn't wear them; (4) sequential development and its expression in body management, fine motor skills, communications, self-care, social interaction with adults and children, and the characteristics of play; (5) integration of family members into the program at some level to contribute to the maintenance of a positive parent-child relationship; and (6) the child's initial and ongoing adjustment to the program.

Pediatricians should have an increasing role in addressing the needs of their own patients who are in day care programs, particularly those children who may be at risk for adapting poorly or who may need special considerations. They should be knowledgeable about the variety of child care settings available in their communities. Pediatricians who are aware of the resources in their communities and who have the skills to recommend a good program, to provide a useful health profile of the child and family, and to be receptive to the concerns of members of the day care program staff will contribute immeasurably to their patients' well-being and successful participation in the day care program.

COMMITTEE ON EARLY CHILDHOOD, ADOPTION AND
DEPENDENT CARE, 1982-1984
Selma R. Deitch, MD, Chairman
David L. Chadwick, MD
Thomas Coleman, MD
Donna O'Hare, MD
Jean Pakter, MD
Burton Sokoloff, MD
George G. Sterne, MD
Virginia Wagner, MD

Liaison Representatives
Elaine Schwartz, Children's Bureau, OHD, DHHS
Helen Felitto, Child Welfare League of America
Jeanne Hunzeker, DSW, Child Welfare League of America
Kenneth Grundfast, MD, Section on Otolaryngology

Consultant
Susan Aronson, MD

APPENDIX I.2

CHILD DAY CARE TERMS FOR THE HEALTH PROFESSIONAL

AFDC:

Aid to Families with Dependent Children, provided under Title IVA of the Social Security Act, provides assistance to eligible families to help preserve, rehabilitate, reunite, and strengthen the family. AFDC mothers in work or training are allowed up to $160.00 per child for child care (1984).

Age Groupings:

These may vary from state to state.

Infant .... 6 weeks to 15 months

Toddler .... 16 months to 30 months

Preschool .... 31 months to 5 years

Primary school .... 6 years to 8 years

Intermediate school .... 9 years to 12 years

Child Care Centers (Day Care Centers, Child Development Centers):

Provide care for more than ten children, often in a church, community center, or school. Most are licensed for children 2½ to 6 years, although care for children from 6 weeks to 2½ years is becoming more available. A center provides a planned curriculum geared to the physical, intellectual, and social needs of the children, giving attention to individual differences. A center is usually open from 6:00 AM to 6:00

PM. Most children attending centers have parents who work or attend school full time. (A license is required but standards vary from state to state.)

Child Care Facility:

Any facility other than a child's home where a person or persons other than family members provide care for a child less than 24 hours a day.

Child Care Food Program:

Provides federal funding for meals served in nonresidential day care centers and family day care homes. The program benefits are targeted for preschool children from low-income families; however, all children attending participating day care facilities receive the benefits of the Child Care Food Program. This program is authorized by Section 17 of the National School Lunch Act, and is administered through the United States Department of Agriculture, Food and Nutrition Service.

Child Development Training:

Child development training includes courses that are relevant to care of children. It may include psychology, early childhood education, infant development, curriculum development, cognitive and effective development, and administrative courses.

Children:

a) Persons 12 years of age or under
b) Children of migrant workers 15 years of age and under

c) Mentally or physically handicapped persons, as defined by the state, enrolled in an institution or a child care facility serving a majority of persons 18 years of age and under.

Children with Disabilities:

Children with disabilities are those who do not function according to age-appropriate expectations in the areas of effective, cognitive, communicative, perceptual-motor, physical, or social development, to such an extent that they require special help, program adjustments, and related services, on a regular basis, in order to function in an adaptive manner. Examples of such children with disabilities may include children who exhibit
• A developmental delay
• A neurologically based condition such as mental retardation, cerebral palsy, autism, epilepsy, or other condition closely related to mental retardation or requiring treatment similar to that required by mentally retarded children
• Cultural familial mental retardation
• A genetic disorder or physiological condition usually associated with mental retardation
• Social/emotional maladjustment
• A physical disability such as a visual impairment, hearing impairment, speech or language impairment, or a physical handicap

Day Care Center Staff Definitions:

The following positions are usually found in large day care centers.

Director: Person responsible for all aspects of the operation of the day care center (e.g., administrative duties, staff supervision and training, recordkeeping, program planning, budgeting, and liaison with state and local agencies).

Teacher: Responsible for planning and implementing the program of the day care center (e.g., plans and conducts daily program activities, prepares program materials, and supervises and trains other staff). This person has direct child contact. Other titles used to designate persons with these responsibilities: teacher-director, head teacher, and lead teacher.

Assistant Teacher: Works with the guidance of the teacher and director to carry out the program of the center.

Child Care Assistant: Assists the teacher or assistant teacher with all the aspects of the planned program. Other titles may include aide, or child care aide.

Family Day Care:

Involves the care of six or fewer children in the caregiver's home. The emphasis is on care for children in the natural setting of a family. Some family day care and group family day care homes offer evening care, second and third shift care, part-time, drop-in, and special needs care. (A license is usually required, depending on the state.)

Family Day Care Consortium or Satellite Program:

Family day care homes operating under the sponsorship of a central administration that processes eligibility and makes placements in the family day care homes. Training of the caregivers can be an additional benefit as part of a satellite program.

FIDCR:

In 1967, amendments to the Federal Economic Opportunity Act established an interagency task force including representatives from the Department of Labor and the Office of Economic Opportunity, Department of Health, Education and Welfare, which developed the Federal Interagency Day Care Requirements (FIDCR) as a "common set of program standards and regulations" for federally funded day care. These standards, enacted in 1968 and slightly amended by Title

XX, cover a number of program characteristics: staff/child ratios and the size of the group; suitability and safety of facilities; the provision of social health and nutritional services; staff training and parent involvement; administrative coordination and program evaluation. In 1974, through Title XX, the Secretary of HEW was required to evaluate the "appropriateness" of FIDCR. In 1981, these regulations were eliminated; licensing is now only regulated through the states.

Group Family Day Care:

Involves the care of up to ten children plus two school-aged children in the caregiver's home. This option keeps the natural setting of a family and still offers the benefit of socializing with a larger group of children. (A license is usually required, depending on the state.)

Head Start:

Federal funding provided to establish and maintain a preschool readiness program for deprived or disadvantaged children.

Informal In-Home Care:

Children cared for in the provider's home. Such providers might include relatives, neighbors, or others who regard child care as a business.

In-Home Care:

Involves the care of the children of one family by someone who is not a member of that family, either in the children's home or the caregiver's home. The caregiver's children may be included in this arrangement. (A license is not required if only one other family besides the caregiver's is involved.)

Latch-key Programs:

This term comes from the days when most children of working parents wore their house keys around their necks on a string or chain and let themselves into their homes before their parents returned from work. Latch-key is care provided for school-aged children before and after school hours.

Licensed Capacity:

Maximum number of children who can be in a center at a given time.

Licensed Family Day Care:

Family day care providers are licensed by the county, city, or state to care for a specific number of children, including their own preschoolers under the age of six, in the provider's home. Licensing insures that the provider is trained, that there is a proper provider/child ratio, and that the provider's home is adequate for the health and safety of the child.

Montessori:

An educational philosophy based on the ideas and methods of Maria Montessori, sometimes used in day care centers. Its focus is a structured, individualized approach, employing special materials.

Night Care Program:

A day care center program providing care for any child between the hours of 7:00 PM and 7:00 AM in which the parents desire the child to sleep.

Parent Cooperative:

A nonprofit child care program that is governed by a board of at least 70% parent-users of the program. Parents generally work as caregivers in the program.

Proprietary Center:

A privately or publicly owned, for-profit center or facility.

Provider:

Provider is a public or private organization or individual who, for profit or not for profit, delivers day care service for children, either directly or through contract.

Sliding Scale:

Fees based on ability to pay according to family size and income level.

Slot:

One space for one child in a facility.

Tax Reduction and Simplification Act of 1977:

This Act made special provisions for family day care providers, allowing them greater ability to take deductions on their residence as a business expense.

Tax Reform Act of 1976:

A measure which eliminated the Federal income tax deduction for child and dependent care expenses and replaces it with a tax credit which is subtracted from the amount of taxes owed.

Title XX:

The section of the Social Security Act which, since 1975, has granted funds to the states for the provision of coordinated social services (including day care) to low-income individuals and families. Its goals are promoting self-support, preventing neglect of children, and reducing inappropriate institutional care. Title XX is now called the Title XX Social Services Block Grant. Each state decides how much of these block grant allocations should be used for child care. Each state also decides the level of income eligibility for services.

WIN:

Work Incentive Program, provided under Title IVC of the Social Security Act, provides training and employment services to individuals over 16 receiving AFDC or living in the same household as an AFDC recipient. AFDC mothers with school-aged children are required to take part in this program if they are not working. Mothers of preschool children who wish to work can receive similar services through the NON-WIN program. Child care subsidies are usually provided for program participants.

Adapted from:
Medical Terms for the Child Day Care Professional and Child
Day Care Terms for the Health Professional
Minnesota Department of Health
June 1984

State of New Hampshire
Department of Health & Welfare
Division of Public Health Services
Bureau of Child Care Standards
and Licensing

CHILD HEALTH FORM

To be completed by Parent or Guardian:

	Date of Birth	Sex
Child's Name		

Child's Address

We/I _____ give permission to obtain or release necessary health information on the above child.

_____
(Signature of Parent or Guardian)

Please return to: _____

This information will be held confidential and will be used only for the benefit of this child.

To be completed by Physician:

HISTORY

A. Prenatal, perinatal and postnatal development: Any significant findings that could influence this child's adaptations to a child care setting (i.e., physical handicap, sensory loss, developmental irregularities)?

B. Any chronic illness that may require regular medication, particularly observations or precautions in a child care setting (e.g., recurrent ear infections, seizure disorder, allergies)?

C. Any hospitalizations, operations, or special tests of which a child care provider should be aware?

D. Pertinent family, social or health characteristics?

E. Immunization and infectious disease history:

	Date of Illness	Date of Immun.	Date of Boosters
Diphtheria			
Pertussis			
Tetanus			
Polio, Oral			
Polio, Salk			
Measles			
Mumps			
Rubella			
Chicken Pox			
Scarlet Fever			
HBPV			

Tests:	Date	Method	Result
TB			
Vision			
Hearing			
Speech			

	Date	Method
Hbg/Hct		
Urine		
Lead		
Other		

HEALTH ASSESSMENT

Form #1 continued

Physical Exam:

Height: _____ Percentile: _____ Weight: _____ Percentile: _____

Head Circumference: _____ Percentile: _____ Blood Pressure: _____

Check (✓) Each Line	Normal	Abnormal	Needs Follow-up	Not Examined
Skin/Scalp				
Nutrition				
Neurolog & Muscular				
Orthopedic & Spine				
Eyes				
Ears				
Speech				

Check (✓) Each Line	Normal	Abnormal	Needs Follow-up	Not Examined
Nose, Throat, Mouth				
Teeth & Gums				
Glands inc. Thyroid				
Chest, Breasts				
Heart, Lungs				
Abdomen				
Genitalia				

Temperament:

☐ Easy-going   ☐ Average   ☐ Difficult

Comments:

Assessment of Physical Development:

A. Estimate of level of maturation:

a. Infancy (0-2 yrs.)   Early: _____ Mid: _____ Late: _____
b. Mid-Preschool (2-4 yrs.)   Early: _____ Mid: _____ Late: _____
c. Preschool (4-6 yrs.)   Early: _____ Mid: _____ Late: _____
d. School-age (6-10 yrs.)   Early: _____ Mid: _____ Late: _____
e. Adolescent (11-18 yrs.)   Early: _____ Mid: _____ Late: _____

B. Estimate of functional capacity:

	Delayed for Develop. Phase	Consistent with Develop. Phase	Advanced for Develop. Phase	Comments
Gross Motor:				
Fine Motor:				
Language Skills:				
Social Skills:				
Emotional:				

C. Impression of child's present state of health:

D. Recommendations regarding:

  a. Medical needs:

  b. Developmental needs:

  c. Family support:

Physician's Signature: _____ Date of Exam: _____

Date of Next Scheduled Exam: _____

This form was designed expressly for child care use in conjunction with the New Hampshire Pediatric Society. 1980.

APPENDIX II.1
Form #2

Pennsylvania Dept. of Health & Welfare, Harrisburg

CHILD HEALTH APPRAISAL
Child Day Care Centers
Group Day Care Homes
Family Day Care Homes

CHILD'S NAME (Last, First, MI)	BIRTHDATE	TELEPHONE NO.	DATE OF EXAM
CHILD'S ADDRESS			

1. REVIEW OF HEALTH HISTORY

2. MEDICAL INFORMATION PERTINENT TO DIAGNOSIS AND TREATMENT IN CASE OF EMERGENCY

3. SPECIAL INSTRUCTIONS TO PROVIDER REGARDING ANY MEDICATION REQUIRED DURING DAY CARE HOURS

4. RECOMMENDED MODIFICATIONS OR LIMITATIONS OF CHILD'S ACTIVITIES OR DIET (e.g. allergies, etc.)

5. VISION (Acuity) ☐ Normal ☐ Abnormal
6. HEARING (audiometry or equiv.) ☐ Normal ☐ Abnormal

7. GROWTH MEASUREMENT
Ht. ___" ___ Percentile Wt. ___ lbs. ___ Percentile Head Circ. ___" ___ Percentile

8. DENTAL SCREENING	YES	NO
Caries		
Missing Permanent Teeth		
Oral Infection		
Protrusion		

9. MEDICAL	Normal	Abnormal	MEDICAL (Cont'd.)	Normal	Abnormal
Eyes			Abdomen		
Ears, Nose			Genitalia, Breasts		
Mouth, Throat			Extremities Joints		
Lungs			Spine		
Cardio-Vascular			Skin, Lymph Nodes		

10. HGB

HGB □ Normal □ Abnormal   GM or HCT □ Normal □ Abnormal %

| 11. BLOOD PRESSURE | □ Normal □ Abnormal | 12. DEVELOPMENTAL APPRAISAL Is child progressing normally with age or group? | □ YES □ NO | Denver Developmental: | □ NORMAL □ ABNORMAL |

13. IMMUNIZATIONS

DTP: Diphtheria Tetanus-Pertussis	Date	Trivalent Oral Polio Vaccine	Date	Other	Date
1st (2 months)		1st (2 months)		Measles (15 months or older)	
2nd (4 months)		2nd (4 months)		Mumps (15 months or older)	
3rd (6 months)		3rd (18 months)		Rubella (15 months or older)	
Booster		4th (4-6 years)		H. Influenzae type b (24-60 months)	
Booster					

14. RECOMMEND FURTHER MEDICAL TESTS OR EXAMINATIONS ON THE FOLLOWING:

□ VISION □ HEARING

□ GROWTH □ DENTAL

□ HGB □ BLOOD PRESSURE

□ HEAD CIRCUMFERENCE □ IMMUNIZATION (specify)

□ MEDICAL (specify)

□ DEVELOPMENTAL PROGRESS (explain)

PHYSICIAN'S SIGNATURE	DATE	PRINTED NAME OF PHYSICIAN
PHYSICIAN'S ADDRESS		TELEPHONE NUMBER

APPENDIX II.2

Sample Program Medication Administration Policy

1. Reasons for administration of medication in day care include
   - When medication dosage cannot be adjusted to exclude hours when the child is in day care.
   - When a child has a chronic medical problem (e.g., asthma) which may require urgent administration of a medication.
   - When refusal to administer medication in day care would pose a significant hardship or require absence from day care of a child in the recovery phase of an illness who is otherwise well enough to attend day care (e.g., ear infection after the first day or so).
   - When those in the home environment cannot administer the medication because of time constraints, lack of skill, or stress.
2. Medications which can be safely given in day care include
   - Medications prescribed by a licensed health professional, such as those available over-the-counter, for which written instructions are given to the day care program by a licensed health provider.
   - Medications which staff who are responsible have been trained to administer including oral, topical, rectal, nasal, otic, ophthalmic, and injectable medications.
   - Medications which bear their original prescription label or a manufacturer's label and which are provided in safety-lock containers, transported safely with regard to temperature, light, and other physical storage requirements.
   - Medications for which all the criteria on the program's consent form have been met.
3. The person(s) responsible for administering medication in day care will be the person(s) who
   - Has designated time for medication administration.
   - Has been trained to administer the type of medication by the route as required.

- Will assure safe storage and disposal of medication.
- Has access to locations where medication is stored and medication administration records are kept.
- Is designated on the program's consent form.
- Knows the children to whom the medication is to be given.
- Knows about the potential reactions to the medications to be administered and how to respond to such reactions.
- Knows when and how to contact parents, pharmacists, or health providers to clarify the need and instructions for administration of medication in day care.

4. Medications will be stored
   - In a refrigerator separated from food by being enclosed in a covered container, if refrigeration is required.
   - In a cool, dry, dark, locked enclosure which is inaccessible to children.
   - In an area separate from child care activities, but accessible to the person who administers the medication.

     Example: All medications which require refrigeration will be kept in a sealed plastic container on the bottom shelf of the refrigerator in the kitchen. Any medication which should not be refrigerated will be kept locked in the director's office.

5. Medications will be administered
   - In a location where the child receiving the medication will have relative privacy when the medication is given. If this is not possible, the other children will be reminded that medications are only taken when the caregiving adult administers them.
   - In a location where accidental ingestion by another child is unlikely.
   - Where hand washing facilities are accessible.

6. Procedures which will be used when administering medication include
   - Designation of time(s) at which the medication can be given.
   - Completion of the consent form.
   - Storage of the medication in the designated locations.
   - Administration using the prescribed measuring device and technique.
   - Recording of each dose given by date, time, and amount on the medication administration record available to the parent.

- Disposal of leftover medications by returning the unused portion to the parents, or if the medication is no longer usable, by flushing the medication down the toilet.
- Review of the medication administration policy on an annual basis by
* those in authority (e.g., administrators).
* those affected by the policy (e.g., parents, staff, etc.).
* those with expertise in medication administration (e.g., health consultant).

Prepared by Susan S. Aronson, M.D.

APPENDIX II.3

Medication Checklist

CHILD'S NAME _____ DATE _____

Does the container show	YES	NO
1. The child's full name	___	___
2. Name of medicine	___	___
3. Name of physician prescribing	___	___
4. Schedule of administration	___	___
5. Amount given per dose	___	___
6. Pharmacy's name	___	___
7. Date medication was sold	___	___
Does the container have a childproof cap?	___	___
Was the caregiver notified of the child's need for medication?	___	___
Was the health staff notified?	___	___
Were parents notified?	___	___

Parent Emergency Contact Number for today is _____

When all of the above are YES, then—give medication to staff member to put in the medicine container in the kitchen refrigerator, and place this checklist in the Health Coordinator's (Health Advocate's) mailbox.

If some of the above are NO, then—give medication to staff member to place in the medicine container in the kitchen refrigerator, but understand that the Health Coordinator or the Health Advocate may contact you (the parent) to discuss the missing information and whether we can administer the medication.

_____

Signature of staff person accepting medication

Prepared by Susan S. Aronson, M.D.

APPENDIX II.4

Medication Consent Form

Name of Child _____ Date _____ Room _____
Name of Medication _____ Date prescribed _____
Date last dose due _____

FOR PARENT TO COMPLETE:

I, _____(parent or guardian) give permission to
_____ (name of authorized day care staff)
to administer _____ (dose) of _____(name of medication)
to my child, _____(name of child)
at approximately _____(time[s] dose due) on
_____ (dates and days) for _____
_____ (reason for medication).
Possible side effects to watch for with this medication include:
_____.
The name and phone number of the prescribing physician:
_____

FOR STAFF TO COMPLETE:

Is the permission form (above) completed? _____
Is the medication in a safety cap container? _____
Is the original prescription label on the medication container?
_____
Is the name of child given above on the container? _____

Is the date on prescription current (within the month for antibiotics and within the expiration date for medications which are so labeled; within the year otherwise)? _____

Is the dose, name of drug, frequency of administration given on the label consistent with parental instructions given above? _____

MEDICATION CAN BE ADMINISTERED ONLY IF THE ANSWERS TO ALL QUESTIONS ABOVE ARE "YES."

MEDICATION ADMINISTRATION RECORD

DAY	DATE	DOSE	STAFF SIGNATURE

Prepared by Susan S. Aronson, M.D.

APPENDIX II.5
STAFF HEALTH APPRAISAL

Pennsylvania Dept. of Health & Welfare, Harrisburg
Child Day Care Centers—Group Day Care Homes—Family Day Care Homes

THIS SECTION TO BE COMPLETED BY THE EMPLOYEE

NAME AND ADDRESS OF INDIVIDUAL EXAMINED

NAME OF EMPLOYER	EMPLOYER'S TELEPHONE NO.

EMPLOYER'S ADDRESS

PURPOSE OF EXAMINATION	TYPE OF ACTIVITY IN DAY CARE (Check all applicable)
☐ Initial Employment	☐ Caring for Children ☐ Food Preparation ☐ Driver of Vehicle
☐ Annual Re-examination	☐ Desk Work ☐ Facility Maintenance

THIS SECTION TO BE COMPLETED BY HEALTH PROFESSIONAL WHO DOES HEALTH APPRAISING

PART I—As shown by physical examination, does the individual have:	YES	NO
1. At least 20/40 combined vision, corrected by glasses, if needed?		
2. Normal hearing?		
3. Normal blood pressure?		
4. Normal cardiovascular system?		
5. Normal respiratory system?		
6. Normal skin?		
7. Normal neuro musculoskeletal systems?		
8. Normal endocrine system?		

EXPLAIN ALL "NO" RESPONSES ON REVERSE OF FORM

	YES	NO
PART II—Is the individual free from communicable tuberculosis as shown by:		
9. Negative skin test results within the past two years?		
10. Positive skin test followed by one negative x-ray and an asymptomatic history at this health appraisal?		
EXPLAIN ALL "NO" RESPONSES ON REVERSE OF FORM, GIVING PLAN FOR FOLLOW-UP		
PART III—Does this individual have any of the following medical problems:	YES	NO
11. History of myocardial infarction, angina pectoris, coronary insufficiency?		
12. History of epilepsy?		
13. Diabetes?		
14. Thyroid or other metabolic disorders?		
15. Inadequate immune status (Td, measles, mumps, rubella)?		
16. Need for more frequent health visits or sick days than average for age?		
17. Current drug or alcohol dependency?		
18. Disabling emotional disorder?		
19. Other special medical problem or chronic disease which requires restriction of activity, medication or which might affect his/her work role? If so, specify on reverse of form.		
EXPLAIN ALL "YES" RESPONSES ON REVERSE OF FORM, GIVING PLAN FOR FOLLOW-UP IF ANY		
20. Does this individual have any special medical problems which might interfere with the health of the children or which might prohibit the individual from providing adequate care for the children? If yes, explain on reverse of form.		

NAME AND ADDRESS OF LICENSED PHYSICIAN	TELEPHONE NUMBER
SIGNATURE OF PHYSICIAN	DATE OF EXAMINATION

APPENDIX II.6

Consent For Staff Access To Medical Records

I, _____, give my consent for the following individuals to have access to my child's record while my child is enrolled in _____

Day Care Program:

My child's caregiver _____

The center's social worker _____

The center's medical consultant _____

The Child Care Supervisor _____

The Director _____

I understand that information in my child's record will not be released to any other individuals without my specific written consent.

Signed _____ Date _____

Witnessed _____

Prepared by Susan S. Aronson, M.D.

APPENDIX II.7

Collecting and Storing Breast Milk

Use any plastic or glass container that can be sterilized. A wide-mouth jar is convenient for collecting and chilling the milk. A plastic or glass baby bottle is often used to store milk in the freezer, so it can be used directly for feeding the baby.

Anything that touches the milk *must* be sterilized—the jar to collect the milk, the baby bottle or other container used for storing the milk.

Put all containers, washed and rinsed, into a pan, cover with cold water, and put on the pan's lid. Bring to a boil, boil for five minutes and turn off the heat. Drain off the water by using the lid. Leave the jars in the pan until needed.

Do not touch the inside part of any sterilized container.

To Collect Milk:

1. Wash the hands with soap and water. Open the clothing so that the entire breast is exposed.
2. Have the containers sterilized and ready to use.
3. Massage the breast and then hand express milk into a sterilized jar.
4. Chill the milk *immediately* in the refrigerator. Milk can be kept for 24 to 48 hours in the refrigerator.
5. If the milk won't be used within 24 hours, pour the chilled milk into another sterilized container in the freezer. A baby bottle is convenient.
6. Milk can be collected an ounce (or less) at a time. Add the new chilled milk to the already frozen milk as a new layer. The milk will look layered.
7. A mother who is collecting the milk for times when she goes out should freeze the milk in amounts that are right for one feeding each. Never fill any container to the very top—allow room for the milk to expand as it freezes. Put 3½ oz. in a 4-oz. bottle for a young baby. Put more ounces in a larger bottle for an older baby.

8. Milk can be kept frozen for months. *Do not defrost* until just before using.

9. When the milk is to be fed to the baby, take the container from the freezer and hold under cold, then warmer water and shake gently. Heat to body temperature in a pan of water.

10. Discard any defrosted milk that the baby does not take.

Answers to Some Frequently Asked Questions:

What does breast milk look like?

It looks thin and watery and sometimes has a yellow or bluish color. It does *not* look like homogenized cows' milk.

How much milk can be expressed at one time?

Never as much as a baby would be able to nurse out. When the colostrum or "first milk" is still in the breasts, often only a few drops can be expressed. Later more can be expressed. Women who do a lot of expressing are able to get more milk out.

When the milk will no longer squirt out, but only comes out in an occasional drop, it's time to stop the massaging and expressing for the time being.

What about expressing milk from engorged breasts?

It's a good idea to hand express a little milk to try to soften the area around the nipple. This makes the nipple stand out so that it is easier for the baby to grasp with his/her mouth. It's better to do this *before* the breasts get too full.

To express milk from engorged breasts: Stand under a warm shower with the back toward the shower and let the water run over the shoulders and breasts, or use warm compresses on the breasts instead of massage (which would be uncomfortable on engorged breasts). Then, very gently, hand express a little milk.

What about going out for a few hours?

Either formula or expressed milk can be left for the baby. If breast milk is used, leave a bottle in the freezer with the amount needed for each feeding that will be missed.

Hand expressing for comfort may be necessary if several hours go by. After returning home, nurse the baby to help empty the breasts and prevent breast problems. The baby sitter can be instructed not to feed the baby right before this time.

Does it matter how often hand expression is done?

Hand expression can build up the milk supply. Whether by nursing or expressing, the more milk removed today, the more milk the breasts will produce tomorrow. Don't hand express *a lot* one day (and build up the supply), and then remove none the next day.

What about when the baby can't nurse but will resume nursing later?

Massage and hand express *enough* to keep up the milk supply—about every three hours in the daytime. Continue expressing by hand until the milk no longer sprays from the nipple.

The supply will no doubt decrease somewhat but can be built up again when the baby resumes nursing.

What about working mothers?

Some working mothers express on the job and chill enough milk for the next day's feedings. Others do not have the time or use of a refrigerator, and only hand express if they need to for comfort. Expressing can prevent overfullness and possible breast problems. Breast problems include cracked nipples, engorged breasts, the occasional plugged duct and the rare abcess.

During the first day(s) at work many women are surprised by how much milk they have. Even women who do not want to save the milk may need to hand express for a few days until their breasts adjust and produce less milk. Hand expressing *some* milk, but not emptying the breasts as the baby would, will result in the milk supply decreasing.

What about full breasts during or after weaning?

The more gradual the weaning, the less fullness there is. If the breasts feel full, hand express some milk for comfort and to prevent breast problems.

What about using disposable nurser bags?

Some women use these successfully, but the bags were not made for freezing and have been known to split open. A common mistake is putting on a twist tie tightly to close the bag without allowing room for the milk to expand. Then the bag may break.

For individual questions, consult your physician.

Excerpted from a pamphlet by:
   Health Education Associates
   520 School House Lane
   Willow Grove, PA 19090

APPENDIX II.8

MEAL PATTERNS

	1-3 years	3-6 years	6-12 years
BREAKFAST			
MILK	½ CUP	¾ CUP	1 CUP
JUICE OR FRUIT OR VEGETABLE	¼ CUP	½ CUP	½ CUP
BREAD OR BREAD ALTERNATE OR	½ SLICE	½ SLICE	1 SLICE
CEREAL	¼ CUP	⅓ CUP	¾ CUP
LUNCH OR SUPPER			
MILK	½ CUP	¾ CUP	1 CUP
MEAT OR POULTRY OR FISH OR	1 OZ.	1½ OZS.	2 OZS.
CHEESE OR	1 OZ.	1½ OZS.	2 OZS.
EGGS OR	1	1	1
PEANUT BUTTER OR	2 TBLS.	3 TBLS.	4 TBLS.
DRIED BEANS AND PEAS	¼ CUP	⅜ CUP	½ CUP
FRUITS (2 OR MORE) OR VEGETABLES (2 OR MORE) OR FRUITS & VEGETABLES TO TOTAL	¼ CUP	½ CUP	¾ CUP
BREAD OR BREAD ALTERNATE OR	½ SLICE	½ SLICE	1 SLICE
ENRICHED PASTA AND GRAINS	¼ CUP	¼ CUP	½ CUP
SNACK			
SELECT 2 OF THE 4 COMPONENTS: MILK, WHOLE, SKIM, LOW-FAT	½ CUP	½ CUP	1 CUP
FRUIT OR VEGETABLE OR JUICE	½ CUP	½ CUP	¾ CUP
BREAD OR CEREAL OR ALTERNATE	½ SLICE	½ SLICE	1 SLICE
OR ENRICHED PASTA AND GRAINS	¼ CUP	¼ CUP	½ CUP
MEAT OR POULTRY OR FISH OR	½ OZ.	½ OZ.	1 OZ.
CHEESE OR	½ OZ.	½ OZ.	1 OZ.
EGGS OR	½ EGG	½ EGG	1 EGG
PEANUT BUTTER OR	1 TBLS.	1 TBLS.	2 TBLS.
DRIED BEANS & PEAS	⅛ CUP	⅛ CUP	¼ CUP

CNETP Connecticut Nutrition Education and Training Program
Department of Nutritional Sciences
College of Agriculture and Natural Resources
University of Connecticut and State Department of Education
Child Nutrition Programs

APPENDIX II.9

Checklist #1

A DAY CARE CHECKLIST FOR PARENTS

Reprinted from *A Parent's Guide to Day Care*, U.S. Department of Health and Human Services, Office of Human Development Services, Administration for Children, Youth and Families, DHHS Publication No. (OHDS) 80-30254.

This checklist is designed to help you decide what things about a day care arrangement are most important to you and your family. It can also help you make sure your child's arrangement offers the things you believe are important.

Read through the checklist and circle those items you want the arrangement to provide. Then, when you talk to a possible caregiver or visit a home or center, decide whether the arrangement offers those things. Just check "yes" or "no." Use the checked-off list to help you make a decision.

Remember, this checklist tries to be as complete as possible. Not everything will apply to your family's situation. Look at the headlines in the lefthand column to see what you should read and what you can skip.

DOES YOUR CHILD'S CAREGIVER ...

For All Children

	Yes	No
Appear to be warm and friendly?	____	____
Seem calm and gentle?	____	____
Seem to have a sense of humor?	____	____
Seem to be someone with whom you can develop a relaxed, sharing relationship?	____	____

Seem to be someone your child will enjoy
   being with?   _____ _____

Seem to feel good about herself and
   her job?   _____ _____

Have child-rearing attitudes and methods
   that are similar to your own?   _____ _____

Treat each child as a special person?   _____ _____

Understand what children can and want to
   do at different stages of growth?   _____ _____

Have the right materials and equipment on
   hand to help them learn and grow mentally
   and physically?   _____ _____

Patiently help children solve their
   problems?   _____ _____

Provide activities that encourage children
   to think things through?   _____ _____

Encourage good health habits, such as
   washing hands before eating?   _____ _____

Talk to the children and encourage them
   to express themselves through words?   _____ _____

Encourage children to express themselves
   in creative ways?   _____ _____

Have art and music supplies suited to
   the ages of all children in care?   _____ _____

Seem to have enough time to look after
   all the children in her care?   _____ _____

Help your child to know, accept, and
   feel good about him- or herself?   _____ _____

Help your child become independent in ways
   you approve?   _____ _____

Help your child learn to get along with and
   respect other people, no matter what their
   backgrounds are?   _____ _____

Provide a routine and rules the children
   can understand and follow?   _____ _____

Accept and respect your family's
   cultural values?   _____ _____

Take time to discuss your child with you
   regularly?   _____ _____

Have previous experience or training in
   working with children?   _____ _____

Have a yearly physical exam and TB test?   _____ _____

And If You Have an Infant or Toddler (Birth to Age 3)

	Yes	No
Seem to enjoy cuddling your baby?	___	___
Care for your baby's physical needs such as feeding and diapering?	___	___
Spend time holding, playing with, talking to your baby?	___	___
Provide stimulation by pointing out things to look at, touch, and listen to?	___	
Provide care you can count on so your baby can learn to trust her and feel important?	___	___
Cooperate with your efforts to toilet train your toddler?	___	___
"Child-proof" the setting so your toddler can crawl or walk safely and freely?	___	___
Realize that toddlers want to do things for themselves and help your child to learn to feed and dress him- or herself, go to the bathroom, and pick up his or her own toys?	___	___
Help your child learn the language by talking with him or her, naming things, reading aloud, describing what she is doing, and responding to your child's words?	___	___

And If Your Child Is a Preschooler (Aged 3 to 5 or 6)

	Yes	No
Plan many different activities for your child?	___	___
Join in activities herself?	___	___
Set consistent limits which help your child gradually learn to make his or her own choices?	___	___
Recognize the value of play and encourage your child to be creative and use his or her imagination?	___	___
Help your child feel good about him- or herself by being attentive, patient, positive, warm, and accepting?	___	___
Allow your child to do things for him- or herself because she understands children can learn from their mistakes?	___	___

Help your child increase his or her vocabulary
   by talking with him or her, reading
   aloud, and answering questions? _____ _____

And If Your Child Is of School Age (Aged 6 to 14)

	Yes	No
Give your child supervision and security but also understand his or her growing need for independence?	___	___
Set reasonable and consistent limits?	___	___
At the same time, allow your child to make choices and gradually take responsibility?	___	___
Understand the conflict and confusion that growing children sometimes feel?	___	___
Help your child follow through on projects, help with homework, and suggest interesting things to do?	___	___
Listen to your child's problems and experiences?	___	___
Respect your child when he or she expresses new ideas, values, or opinions?	___	___
Cooperate with you to set clear limits and expectations about behavior?	___	___
Understand the conflicts and confusion older school-age children feel about sex, identity, and pressure to conform?	___	___
Provide your child with a good adult image to admire and copy?	___	___

DOES THE DAY CARE HOME OR CENTER HAVE...

For All Children

	Yes	No
An up-to-date license, if one is required?	___	___
A clean and comfortable look?	___	___
Enough space indoors and out so all the children can move freely and safely?	___	___
Enough caregivers to give attention to all of the children in care?	___	___

Enough furniture, play things, and other
    equipment for all the children in care?   ____ ____

Equipment that is safe and in good repair?   ____ ____

Equipment and materials that are suitable
    for the ages of the children in care?   ____ ____

Enough room and cots or cribs so the
    children can take naps?   ____ ____

Enough clean bathrooms for all the
    children in care?   ____ ____

Safety caps on electrical outlets?   ____ ____

A safe place to store medicines, household
    cleansers, poisons, matches, sharp
    instruments, and other dangerous items?   ____ ____

An alternate exit in case of fire?   ____ ____

A safety plan to follow in emergencies?   ____ ____

An outdoor play area that is safe, fenced,
    and free of litter?   ____ ____

Enough heat, light, and ventilation?   ____ ____

Nutritious meals and snacks made with the
    kinds of food you want your child to eat?   ____ ____

A separate place to care for sick children
    where they can be watched?   ____ ____

A first aid kit?   ____ ____

Fire extinguishers?   ____ ____

Smoke detectors?   ____ ____

Covered radiators and protected heaters?   ____ ____

Strong screens or bars on windows
    above the first floor?   ____ ____

And If You Have an Infant or Toddler (Birth to Age 3)

                  Yes   No

Gates at tops and bottoms of stairs?   ____ ____

A potty chair or special toilet seat in the
    bathroom?   ____ ____

A clean and safe place to change diapers?   ____ ____

Cribs with firm mattresses covered in
    heavy plastic?   ____ ____

Separate crib sheets for each baby in care?   ____ ____

And If Your Child Is a Preschooler (Aged 3 to 5 or 6)

                  Yes   No

A stepstool in the bathroom so your
    pre-schooler can reach the sink and toilet?   ____ ____

And If Your Child Is of School Age (Aged 6 to 14)

	Yes	No
A quiet place to do homework?	___	___
Places to store personal belongings?	___	___

ARE THERE OPPORTUNITIES ...

For All Children

	Yes	No
To play quietly and actively, indoors and out?	___	___
To play alone at times and with friends at other times?	___	___
To follow a schedule that meets young children's need for routine but that is flexible enough to meet the needs of each child?	___	___
To use materials and equipment that help children learn new physical skills and control and exercise their muscles?	___	___
To learn to get along, to share, and to respect themselves and others?	___	___
To learn about their own and others' cultures through art, music, books, songs, games, and other activities?	___	___
To speak both English and their family's native language?	___	___
To watch special programs on television that have been approved by you?	___	___

And If You Have an Infant or Toddler (Birth to Age 3)

	Yes	No
To crawl and explore safely?	___	___
To play with objects and toys that help infants to develop their senses of touch, sight, and hearing (for example, mobiles, mirrors, cradle gyms, crib toys, rattles, things to squeeze and roll, pots and pans, nesting cups, different sized boxes)?	___	___

To take part in a variety of activities
    that are suited to toddlers' short attention
    spans (for example, puzzles, cars,
    books, outdoor play equipment for active
    play; modeling clay, clocks, boxes,
    containers, for creative play)?   ____   ____

And If Your Child Is a Preschooler (Aged 3 to 5 or 6)

                                                        Yes   No

To play with many different toys and
    equipment that enable preschoolers to use
    their imaginations (for example, books,
    musical instruments, costumes)?   ____   ____
To choose their own activities, for at
    least part of the day?   ____   ____
To visit nearby places of interest, such
    as the park, the library, the fire house,
    a museum?   ____   ____

And If Your Child Is of School Age (Aged 6 to 14)

                                                        Yes   No

To practice their skills (for example,
    sports equipment, musical instruments,
    drama activities, craft projects)?   ____   ____
To be with their own friends after school?   ____   ____
To do homework?   ____   ____
To use a variety of materials and equipment
    including: art materials, table games,
    sports equipment, books, films, and
    records?   ____   ____
To use community facilities such as a
    baseball field, a swimming pool, a
    recreation center?   ____   ____

APPENDIX II.9

Checklist #2

A QUESTIONNAIRE FOR PARENTS TO USE WHEN EVALUATING CHILD CARE

Make a list of the child care facilities you wish to explore. Bring this sheet with you to see how many of the questions are answered YES. Looks may be deceiving—be objective! This should make your choice easier and more rational. What is important to you in terms of your child's mental and physical growth? Don't do your searching at the last minute!

NAME OF FACILITY _____

DATE VISITED _____

1. Is the child care facility licensed? (Ask to see the current license.)   YES   NO
2. Is the location convenient to your home?   YES   NO
3. Is your initial reaction to the facility positive? (Trust your feelings.)   YES   NO
4. Are all the costs written out and easily available for you to read?   YES   NO
5. Is there extra after-hours care available in case of emergency or inability to reach the facility at your prearranged pick-up time?   YES   NO
6. Can you visit the facility during regular operating hours before registering your children in the program?   YES   NO
7. Is the number of adult caregivers sufficient for the children present?   YES   NO
8. Do the caregivers TEACH in addition to seeing after the usual basic needs?   YES   NO
9. Does the staff appear to enjoy caring for the children?   YES   NO

10. Is the staff at eye level with the children when engaged in activities with them or do they stand above them when playing or instructing them?   YES   NO

11. Does the facility appear to be clean?   YES   NO

12. Will the staff allow you to examine the entire premises?   YES   NO

13. Can parents visit whenever they wish? (Restricted visiting times are improper.)   YES   NO

14. Do the children already in the facility appear happy/sad? (Circle one.)   YES   NO

15. Do the adults and children interact?   YES   NO

16. Does there appear to be enough space for the number of children present?   YES   NO

17. Is there a sleeping (quiet) area large enough to accommodate all the children?   YES   NO

18. Are beds, hammocks, or mattresses available to sleep on?   YES   NO

19. Does each child have a specific place for his/her own belongings?   YES   NO

20. Are all the medicines and poisonous substances LOCKED UP? (Ask to check.)   YES   NO

21. Is a list of the meals/snacks readily available (Ask to see it.)   YES   NO

22. Are the meals/snacks nutritious and balanced?   YES   NO

23. Are infants fed lying down? (Bottle propping is unhealthy.)   YES   NO

24. Can your child get a special diet if necessary?   YES   NO

25. Are all the toys to play with at the facility chosen with safety in mind?   YES   NO

26. Are there many toys present for your child's particular age?   YES   NO

27. Is there an outside area available for play activities?   YES   NO

28. Does the outside area appear to be planned for safe playing? (Hard surfaces and rocks, high climbers, slides, swings are dangerous.)   YES   NO

29. Is there a written plan for play activities?
(Ask to see it.)   YES NO
30. Are inside *and* outside play supervised all
the time?   YES NO
31. Are the older and younger children playing
together or in their own age groups? (Mixed
play leads to a higher percentage of
accidents.)   YES NO
32. Is a large part of planned activities
television viewing? (This is not
recommended and may be harmful if
programming is not carefully supervised.)   YES NO
33. Are the parents encouraged to become
involved in any activities?   YES NO
34. Are learning experiences available through
the facility for the parents? (Some child care
centers have parenting and other classes
scheduled.)   YES NO
35. Does the staff regularly meet with
individual parents? (Ask how often.)   YES NO
36. Do the caregivers have a written policy
concerning discipline? (Ask to read it.)   YES NO
37. Are there policies for the care of ill
children? (Ask to see them.)   YES NO
38. Is there a holding area for ill children?   YES NO
39. Will the caregivers administer prescribed
medications to your children?   YES NO
40. Is there a physician consultant for the child
care facility?   YES NO
41. Have personnel had training in first aid and
infectious diseases?   YES NO

IF YOU HAVE ANY QUESTIONS, TALK TO YOUR DOC-
TOR ABOUT THEM. GOOD LUCK IN YOUR SEARCH.

Prepared by
Bruce M. Gach, M.D.
Livermore, California
Rev. 10/85

APPENDIX II.9

Checklist #3

INFORMATION ABOUT CHILD CARE

TYPES OF CARE:

Licensed:
  I. Child Care Centers (nursery schools, preschools, infant centers)—provide full- or part-time care. Care is provided in a group setting in a building which has passed licensing standards for child care (community center, church, school, specially designed facility). A maximum of four children under two years of age for each adult caregiver. A maximum of 12 children over two years of age for each adult present.
 II. Family Child Care Homes—provided in homes of caregivers.
     a) Small—six or fewer children including those of the provider. Limited to three children under two years of age if children over two years of age are being cared for at the same time.
     b) Large—seven to 12 children including those of the provider. Another adult assistant must be present at all times.

Nonlicensed:
  I. In-Home Care—provider comes to parent's/child's house (most expensive).
 II. Cooperative or Shared Care—informal agreements between families such as shared baby sitting, child care exchanges, play groups with shared responsibilities and other arrangements. No adult/child ratio required.
III. Family Day Care Homes—provider caring for only one other family including her own. There is no limit to the number of children.

WHAT DOES LICENSING MEAN?

A license only means that the facility and its providers have met health, fire, and safety standards. These are minimal at best. Also, there is a specified staff/child ratio and capacity for the facility which must be maintained. Basic director and teacher qualifications are required. All personnel have been fingerprinted and none have known criminal records. An initial visit to the facility has been completed at the time of licensure by the local Department of Social Services. Another visit will occur on application renewal three years later unless some complaint is brought against the facility. Then the visit is sooner.

HOW DOES A PARENT KNOW IF A FACILITY IS INTELLECTUALLY AND SOCIALLY ADEQUATE FOR HIS OR HER CHILD?

Since licensing does not monitor the program's content or the actual care in the facility, it is up to each parent to evaluate his or her child's care. A child care arrangement should not be considered only a drop-off and pick-up point so a parent may go to work. It may be the child's major contact with socialization and learning during the weekday waking hours. Talk to your children about their day; observe whether they are happy.

WHO CAN HELP PARENTS CHOOSE WHICH CHILD CARE FACILITY IS BEST SUITED FOR THEIR CHILD?

Every county in California, for example, has local Resource and Referral agencies which may be contacted. These "R and Rs" have current information concerning the care available, types of special programs, and possible subsidies to pay for care. They usually list all the licensed facilities, but may have information on some of the nonlicensed care also. The local state Department of Social Services office has a list of licensed facilities only. The telephone numbers for Child Care Resource and Referral or Information and Referral agencies or the Department of Social Services is in the telephone directory. Another excellent source of information is other parents who have or have had their children in local child care facilities. Use the information from all these sources to make your choice.

WHAT SHOULD PARENTS WATCH FOR IN THEIR CHILD IF CONCERNED ABOUT POSSIBLE PROBLEMS AT A CHILD CARE FACILITY? WHAT SHOULD THEY DO IF THEY BELIEVE A PROBLEM EXISTS?

Watch for unwillingness to return to the facility, beyond the usual not wanting to separate from parents; wanting to wear more clothing, especially underclothes; change in usual eating or toilet habits; fear of going to sleep or nightmares for no apparent reason; illness which gets better as the day progresses; not wanting to talk about what was done at the caregivers'; fear of strangers more than usual; other changes you feel are abnormal. If you are concerned, talk to your child and tell him/her that it is all right to tell you about a problem even if someone told them not to talk about it. Look for any marks on the skin which cannot be explained from your observation of the child's activities. If you feel that a problem exists at a facility—licensed or not—contact your local Child Protective Agency listed in your telephone book. You may also contact the local Department of Social Services. The facility will be investigated—it's required by law—although you may not get a personal report of the findings. Expect that you will also be interviewed by an experienced person who has been trained to handle cases similar to yours.

Do NOT go to the provider and confront her or him with your suspicions if you feel a problem exists. This may harm any investigation and possible evidence. Remove your child from that caregiver—you'll never be at ease about that person again. If you have many doubts about whether a problem exists, talk over your concerns with other parents using the same source of care to see if they have similar concerns.

IS THERE SOME SORT OF GOVERNMENTAL HELP TO MEET THE EXPENSES OF CHILD CARE?

There are Federal and State tax credits currently available. Some businesses subsidize child care—ask your employer if such a program is a benefit. Contracting agencies such as the "R and Rs" have various subsidies available. Unfortunately, the list of applicants for these monies is usually filled. Ask to have your name placed on the waiting list.

BRUCE M. GACH, M.D.
Livermore, California

APPENDIX II.9

Checklist #4

HOW TO CHOOSE A GOOD EARLY CHILDHOOD PROGRAM*

What should parents look for in selecting a good early childhood program? The most popular public information brochure from the National Association for the Education of Young Children (NAEYC) has just been rewritten to reflect current research and theory about what is best for young children in group programs. Teachers and program directors also have found it useful for evaluation and staff development. "How to Choose a Good Early Childhood Program" is reprinted in this issue of *Young Children* so that all NAEYC members will know how valuable this information is for parents, the media, decision makers, and our profession.

A good early childhood program can benefit your child, your family, and your community. Your child's educational, physical, personal, and social development will be nurtured in a well-planned program. As a parent, you will feel more confident when your child is enrolled in a suitable program, and the time your family spends together will be more satisfying as a result. Early childhood education plays an important role in supporting families, and strong families are the basis of a thriving community.

If you are thinking about enrolling your child in an early childhood program, you probably have already decided upon some of your basic priorities, such as location, number of hours, cost, and type of care that best suits your child. If you feel that a group program is appropriate, you can obtain a list of licensed programs for young children from your local licensing agency. Then you can call several programs for further information, and arrange to visit the programs that

*Reprinted from: How to Choose a Good Early Childhood Program. National Association for the Education of Young Children (NAEYC), 1834 Connecticut Avenue, N.W., Washington, D.C. 20009. 1 November 1983.

seem best for you and your child so you can talk with teachers, directors, and other parents.

What should you look for in a good early childhood program?

Professionals in early childhood education and child development have found several indicators of good quality care for preschool children. You will especially want to meet the adults who will care for your child—they are responsible for every aspect of the program's operation.

Who will care for your child?

1. **The adults enjoy and understand how young children learn and grow.**

    Are the staff members friendly and considerate to each child?

    Do adult expectations vary appropriately for children of different ages and interests?

    Do the staff members consider themselves to be professionals? Do they read or attend meetings to continue to learn more about how young children grow and develop?

    Do the staff work toward improving the quality of the program, obtaining better equipment, and making better use of the space?

2. **The staff view themselves positively and therefore can continually foster children's emotional and social development.**

    Do the staff help children feel good about themselves, their activities, and other people?

    Do the adults listen to children and talk with them?

    Are the adults gentle while being firm, consistent, and yet flexible in their guidance of children?

    Do the staff members help children learn gradually how to consider others' rights and feelings, to take turns and share, yet also to stand up for personal rights when necessary?

When children are angry or fearful, are they helped to deal with their feelings constructively?

3. **There are enough adults to work with a group and to care for the individual needs of children.**

Are there at least one teacher and an assistant with every group of children?

Are infants in groups of no more than eight children?

Are two- and three-year-old children in groups of no more than 16?

Are four- and five-year-olds in groups of no more than 22 children?

4. **All staff members work together cooperatively.**

Do the staff meet regularly to plan and evaluate the program?

Are they willing to adjust the daily activities for children's individual needs and interests?

5. **Staff observe and record each child's progress and development.**

Do the staff stress children's strengths and show pride in their accomplishments?

Are records used to help parents and staff better understand the child?

Are the staff responsible to parents' concerns about their child's development?

What program activities and equipment are offered?

1. **The environment fosters the growth and development of young children working and playing together.**

Does the center have realistic goals for children?

Are activities balanced between vigorous outdoor play and quiet indoor play?

Are children given opportunities to select activities of interest to them?

Are children encouraged to work alone as well as in small groups?

Are self-help skills such as dressing, toileting, resting, washing, and eating encouraged as children are ready?

Are transition times approached as pleasant learning opportunities?

2. **A good center provides appropriate and sufficient equipment and play materials and makes them readily available.**

   Is there large climbing equipment? Is there an ample supply of blocks of all sizes, wheel toys, balls, and dramatic play props to foster physical development as well as imaginative play?

   Are there ample tools and hands-on materials such as sand, clay, water, wood, and paint to stimulate creativity?

   Is there a variety of sturdy puzzles, construction sets, and other small manipulative items available to children?

   Are children's picture books age-appropriate, attractive, and of good literary quality?

   Are there plants, animals, or other natural science objects for children to care for or observe?

   Are there opportunities for music and movement experiences?

3. **Children are helped to increase their language skills and to expand their understanding of the world.**

   Do the children freely talk with each other and the adults?

   Do the adults provide positive language models in describing objects, feelings, and experiences?

   Does the center plan for visitors or trips to broaden children's understandings through firsthand contacts with people and places?

   Are the children encouraged to solve their own problems, to think independently, and to respond to open-ended questions?

How does the staff relate to your family and the community?

1. **A good program considers and supports the needs of the entire family.**

   Are parents welcome to observe, discuss policies, make suggestions, and participate in the work of the center?

   Do staff members share with parents the highlights of their child's experiences?

Are the staff alert to matters affecting any member of the family which may also affect the child?

Do the staff respect families from varying cultures or backgrounds?

Does the center have written policies about fees, hours, holidays, illness, and other considerations?

2. **A good center is aware of and contributes to community resources.**

Do the staff share information about community recreational and learning opportunities with families?

Do the staff refer family members to a suitable agency when the need arises?

Are volunteers from the community encouraged to participate in the center's activities?

Does the center collaborate with other professional groups to provide the best care possible for children in the community?

Are the facility and program designed to meet the varied demands of young children, their families, and the staff?

1. **The health of children, staff, and parents is protected and promoted.**

Are the staff alert to the health and safety of each child and of themselves?

Are meals and snacks nutritious, varied, attractive, and served at appropriate times?

Do the staff wash hands with soap and water before handling food and after changing diapers? Are children's hands washed before eating and after toileting?

Are surfaces, equipment, and toys cleaned daily? Are they in good repair?

Does each child have an individual cot, mat, or crib?

Are current medical records and emergency information maintained for each child and staff member? Is adequate sick leave provided for staff so they can remain at home when they are ill?

Is at least one staff member trained in first aid? Does the center have a health consultant?

Is the building comfortably warm in cold weather? Are the rooms ventilated with fresh air daily?

2. **The facility is safe for children and adults.**

Are the building and grounds well lighted and free of hazards?

Are furnishings, sinks, and toilets safely accessible to children?

Are toxic materials stored in a locked cabinet?

Are smoke detectors installed in appropriate locations?

Are indoor and outdoor surfaces cushioned with materials such as carpet or wood chips in areas with climbers, slides, or swings?

Does every staff member know what to do in an emergency? Are emergency numbers posted by the telephone?

3. **The environment is spacious enough to accommodate a variety of activities and equipment.**

Are there at least 35 square feet of usable playroom floor space indoors per child and 75 square feet of play space outdoors per child?

Is there a place for each child's personal belongings such as a change of clothes?

Is there enough space so that adults can walk between sleeping children's cots?

If you have remaining questions about how to select a good program, consult an NAEYC Affiliate Group, the early childhood department of a local college, your state licensing agency, or others knowledgeable about early childhood education.

APPENDIX II.9

Checklist #5

POINTS TO THINK ABOUT IN CHOOSING A FAMILY DAY CARE HOME FOR YOUR CHILD

Q. What is a Family Day Care home?

A. It is a home in which children live during day-time hours only. Here they receive care from a motherly person, who is not related to them. They go to their own homes and parents at night.

Q. How many children may be cared for in a Family Day Care home?

A. Not more than two youngsters if they are under two years old, and never more than five children all together.

Q. What kind of person makes a good Family Day Care mother?

A. A friendly, healthy person of good character and reputation.

Q. How about the other members of her family?

A. They should all be healthy, as shown by a recent medical examination report of each one—including a chest X-ray of each adult in the home. Then you are sure that they are in satisfactory physical condition.

Q. What do I look for in a Family Day Care mother?

A. Is she kind and does she like your child? Is she motherly toward all the children who stay with her? Does she understand what each child needs—proper diet, play, rest, etc.?

Q. How can I tell whether this is a good home for my child during the day when I am away from him?

A. Are you comfortable with the Family Day Care mother? Do you like and trust her? Does she ask questions that will help her to understand your child better? Does she agree with you about important things?

Q. How much will I have to pay?

A. There is no set amount. This must be worked out so it

is satisfactory to you and to her. Do not leave your child until you have a clear and definite agreement.

Q. **How do I know whether a home is licensed or approved by the Health Department—or whether it is on the way to getting a license?**

A. Ask the family day care mother. If she has no license or approval, ask her to get in touch with the Health Department.

Q. **What do I look for in the home?**

A. Be sure the home is safe, clean, and in good repair. The rooms should be light, properly heated and well ventilated. Is there space to play, indoors and outdoors? Is there a clean, airy place for a rest? Is the kitchen clean? Is there a refrigerator? Is the bathroom clean? Does it have a toilet, and a wash basin with running hot and cold water?

Q. **What responsibility do I have before I leave my child in a Family Day Care home?**

A. It is most important for you to do the following:

Write down your child's real name, his nick-name (or pet name), and date of birth.

Write down your own name, address, and phone number, and that of your spouse.

Write down the name, address, and telephone number of the doctor or clinic for your child, in case of any emergency.

Write down that you give the Family Day Care mother your permission to take your child to this doctor or clinic in case of an emergency. This is most important for you to do.

Write down the name, address, and phone number of the place where you can be reached during the day.

Give the Family Day Care mother an up-to-date record of a physical examination of your child by a doctor, with any advice or recommendation he or she may have regarding your child.

Tell the Family Day Care mother about your child's eating and sleeping habits, his toilet habits, the things he enjoys, and the things he is afraid of. Help her to know your child. Can he wash and toilet himself? Does he have a favorite toy to go to sleep with?

Q. How can I be most helpful to my child and to the Family Day Care mother?

A. By making one or more visits to the home with your child before you leave him there. Talk to your child naturally and easily so as to be sure he understands and knows he will continue to live with you. Give him time to understand and to become familiar with the new situation. Always be truthful. Do not make any promises you do not expect to keep. Answer his questions.

Q. How long will it take him to become adjusted?

A. This varies greatly and depends on the age of the child and on how comfortable he is in the new home. Give him time to get used to it. If he seems worried or anxious try to stay with him for a time each day. Bring one or several of your child's favorite toys and/or blanket. Talk with the Family Day Care mother each day so you and she can keep each other up-to-date about your youngster.

Q. Will it be upsetting in the beginning?

A. It may be hard in the beginning for all three of you. Try to be understanding, supportive, and patient.

Q. How can I know whether I am making a mistake?

A. See whether the youngster is overcoming his fears about being left and is becoming interested in going. See whether he eats and sleeps well when he is at home. Is his color good? Is he normally active and spry? Does he talk about the things he does and what happens during the day? Does your doctor feel he is O.K.?

Q. If I am worried and unhappy about my child in the Family Day Care home, where can I get help or advice?

A. Perhaps from your husband or someone in your family whose judgment you trust; perhaps from a professional person who works with children and families, like your doctor or minister, or a Department of Health Consultant in the Division of Day Care.

When you have seen your child thrive in his Family Day Care Home, you can be sure you have chosen wisely.

THE DIVISION OF DAY CARE
BUREAU OF CHILD HEALTH
65 Worth Street
New York, NY 10013

APPENDIX II.9

Checklist #6

QUESTIONS AND ANSWERS ABOUT CHILD CARE

The following are questions parents frequently ask about child care:

I feel so guilty about having someone else care for my child. Won't this separation interfere with my child's development and our relationship?

Available evidence indicates that the opposite is true. There are many books, papers, and manuals that support the idea that quality day care services usually enhance child maturation and development and may improve the parent-child relationship.

Is day care harmful to the physical health of my child?

Children in high quality day care compare very favorably with children reared in their own home in terms of physical health. The advantage of early detection and treatment of illness appears to far outweigh the slightly increased possibility of picking up mild infections such as colds and diarrhea. Also, a carefully planned nutrition program can not only improve the health of the child, but also provide nutrition education for both the child and the family.

Is day care harmful to the mental and social development of my child?

Available evidence appears to indicate that children in child care compare very favorably developmentally with children who remain at home with their parents. The benefits of developing cognitive, affective, and social skills through interaction with other children and nonfamily adults in a safe, structured setting supervised by a caring, knowledgeable adult are far greater than the possibility that the child will miss some of the warmth and depth of the parent-child relationship.

Will my child love and respect the caregiver more than me?

There is abundant evidence that children in day care still look to their parents when there are decisions to be made and prefer their parents in times of stress. It is not the amount of time parent and child are together that establishes appropriate bonding and attachment, but rather the quality, security, and predictability of that interaction.

Will a child who attends a day care center or nursery school be bored when he or she goes to school?

All the evidence appears to show that this is not true. The gains children make in emotional, social, and cognitive well-being in quality developmental day care appear to improve their motivation for learning and hence their school performance.

Will the day care center or other caregiver handle my child differently than I do and make it difficult for me to rear my child the way I want to? In short, will my child be brainwashed and alienated from the family?

The best way to avoid this problem is for parents to be involved with their child's care and to communicate with the caregiver. If the differences are too great, a change of setting is advisable.

Friedman DB, Sale JS, Weinstein V: Reprinted with permission from *Child Care and the Family*, National Committee for Prevention of Child Abuse, ISBN 0-937906-39-5, Chicago, IL, 1984

APPENDIX IV.1

Summary Of Clues To Child Abuse

Historical

1. Unexplained or inadequately explained injuries.
2. Changing explanations of injuries.
3. Injuries explained by caregiver(s) as resulting from child behavior impossible for that stage of development.
4. Alleged self-inflicted or third-party inflicted injuries.

Physical

5. Excessive bruising or skin injury, especially in unusual locations.
6. Repeated injuries (even if apparently accidental) and failure to thrive.
7. Typical identifiable lesions (e.g., spiral or chip fractures) or marks (e.g., strap marks or immersion burns).
8. Head and neck (including retinal hemorrhages and subdural hematomas), genital and abdominal visceral injuries.

Behavioral

9. Inexplicable changes in child behavior, including hyper- and hypo-activity, over- and undercompliance, e.g., no selectivity in friendly approach to adults and/or child's claim of mistreatment.
10. Changes in adult attitude toward or behavior in relation to child.
11. Inappropriate behavior of significant adults in interview situation.

12. Delay in seeking medical attention for child, lack of interest in child's medical condition or well-being, and/or refusal or failure to follow appropriate therapeutic recommendations.

Prepared by
Alma S. Friedman, M.S.W. and
David B. Friedman, M.D.

APPENDIX IV.2

Characteristics Of Abusive Adult Family Members

1. Appear dependent and show need of nurturance
   a. Deprivation experiences and/or often abused as children
   b. Negative or poor self-image
2. Fear of relationships
   a. Isolate themselves
   b. Make themselves difficult to like
3. Lack of support systems
   a. Unable to reach out
   b. Never learned to ask for and receive help
4. Marital problems
   a. Choose mate like themselves
   b. Child or children often means of communication
5. Life crises
   a. Unable to control own life
   b. Lack self-control
   c. Impulsive behavior
6. Inability to care for and protect child
   a. See child as "special"
   b. Expectation that child fill adult needs
   c. Inappropriate expectations of normal and handicapped child
   d. Role reversals
   e. Child as extension of self or living through child
7. Lack of nurturing child-rearing practices
   a. Abuse or neglect in adult's childhood
   b. Problem with "inner child of the past"
   c. Confusion of discipline and punishment
   d. Cultural and subcultural punishment child-rearing practices

Prepared by
Alma S. Friedman, MSW and
David B. Friedman, M.D.

APPENDIX V.1

Recommendations For The Immunization Of Caregivers In Child Day Care Centers (Centers For Disease Control 1983)

Immunity to the following diseases is recommended for caregivers in child day care centers:
Diphtheria, tetanus, mumps, measles, poliomyelitis, rubella

A record indicating immunity to these diseases must show the following:

Diphtheria and tetanus:
Completion of a primary series (3 doses) for tetanus and diphtheria; boosters within the past 10 years.

Mumps:
Vaccination with mumps vaccine on or after the first birthday, or
Date of physician-diagnosed mumps disease, or laboratory evidence of immunity.

Measles:
Immunization of individuals born after 1956 (persons born before 1956 are considered immune);
Vaccination with live measles vaccine on or after 15 months of age, or
Date of physician-diagnosed measles disease, or
Laboratory evidence of immunity.

Polio:
Vaccination with a primary series (3 or more doses) of polio vaccine for any caregiver less than 18 years old or still in high school.

Rubella:
Vaccination with rubella vaccine on or after the first birthday, or
Laboratory evidence of immunity.
Immunity to this disease is especially important for women of childbearing age. (A history of rubella disease is not adequate evidence of immunity.)

Measles, mumps, rubella vaccine should be used if a caregiver is thought to be susceptible to more than one component of measles, mumps, and rubella. There is no evidence of adverse reactions following vaccination of individuals who are immune.

APPENDIX V.2

GUIDELINES FOR HEALTH SUPERVISION

Each child and family is unique; therefore these **Guidelines for Health Supervision of Children and Youth**[1] are designed for the care of children who are receiving competent parenting, have no manifestations of any important health problems, and are growing and developing in satisfactory fashion. **Additional visits may become necessary** if circumstances suggest variations from normal. These guidelines represent a consensus by the Committee on Practice and Ambulatory Medicine, in consultation with the membership of the American Academy of Pediatrics through the Chapter Chairmen.

The Committee emphasizes the great importance of **continuity of care** in comprehensive health supervision[2] and the need to avoid **fragmentation of care**[3].

A **prenatal visit** by the parents for anticipatory guidance and pertinent medical history is strongly recommended.

Health supervision should begin with medical care of the newborn in the hospital.

AGE[4]	INFANCY						EARLY CHILDHOOD					LATE CHILDHOOD					ADOLESCENCE			
	By 1 mo.	2 mos.	4 mos.	6 mos.	9 mos.	12 mos.	15 mos.	18 mos.	24 mos.	3 yrs.	4 yrs.	5 yrs.	6 yrs.	8 yrs.	10 yrs.	12 yrs.	14 yrs.	16 yrs.	18 yrs.	20+ yrs.
HISTORY Initial/Interval	●	●	●	●	●	●	●	●	●	●	●	●	●	●	●	●	●	●	●	●
MEASUREMENTS Height and Weight	●	●	●	●	●	●	●	●	●	●	●	●	●	●	●	●	●	●	●	●
Head Circumference	●	●	●	●	●	●														
Blood Pressure										●	●	●	●	●	●	●	●	●	●	●
SENSORY SCREENING Vision	S	S	S	S	S	S	S	S	S	○	○	○	S[5]	S[5]	S[5]	○	○	S	○	S
Hearing	S	S	S	S	S	S	S	S	S	○	○	○	S[5]	S[5]	S[5]	○	S	S	○	S
DEVEL./BEHAV. ASSESSMENT[6]	●	●	●	●	●	●	●	●	●	●	●	●	●	●	●	●	●	●	●	●

PHYSICAL EXAMINATION[7]

PROCEDURES[8]

Hered./Metabolic Screening[9]

Immunization[10]

Tuberculin Test

Hematocrit or Hemoglobin[12]

Urinalysis[13]

ANTICIPATORY GUIDANCE[14]

INITIAL DENTAL REFERRAL[15]

1. Committee on Practice and Ambulatory Medicine, 1981.
2. Statement on Continuity of Pediatric Care, Committee on Standards of Child Care, 1978.
3. Statement on Fragmentation of Pediatric Care, Committee on Standards of Child Health Care, 1978.
4. If a child comes under care for the first time at any point on the Schedule, or if any items are not accomplished at the suggested age, the Schedule should be brought up to date at the earliest possible time.
5. At these points, history may suffice; if problem suggested, a standard testing method should be employed.
6. By history and appropriate physical examination; if suspicious, by specific objective developmental testing.
7. At each visit, a complete physical examination is essential, with infant totally unclothed, older child undressed and suitably draped.
8. These may be modified, depending upon entry point into schedule and individual need.
9. PKU and thyroid testing should be done at about 2 wks. Infants initially screened before 24 hours of age should be rescreened.

Key: ● = to be performed; S = subjective, by history; O = objective, by a standard testing method.

10. Schedule(s) per Report of Committee on Infectious Disease, ed. 20, 1986.
11. The Committee on Infectious Diseases recommends tuberculin testing at 12 months of age and every 1-2 years thereafter. In some areas, tuberculosis is of exceedingly low occurrence and the physician may elect not to retest routinely or to use longer intervals.
12. Present medical evidence suggests the need for reevaluation of the frequency and timing of hemoglobin or hematocrit tests. One determination is therefore suggested during each time period. Performance of additional tests is left to the individual practice experience.
13. Present medical evidence suggests the need for reevaluation of the frequency and timing of urinalyses. One determination is therefore suggested during each time period. Performance of additional tests is left to the individual practice experience.
14. Appropriate discussion and counselling should be an integral part of each visit for care.
15. Subsequent examinations as prescribed by dentist.

N.B.: **Special chemical, immunologic, and endocrine testing are usually carried out upon specific indications.** Testing other than newborn (e.g., inborn errors of metabolism, sickle disease, lead) are discretionary with the physician.

APPENDIX V.3

Immunization Protects Children

Childhood immunization means protection against eight major diseases: poliomyelitis, measles, mumps, rubella (German measles), whooping cough (pertussis), diphtheria, tetanus, and *Haemophilus influenzae* type b infections. Is your child fully protected?

Check the table and ask your pediatrician if your child is up-to-date on vaccines. It could save a life or prevent disability. Measles, mumps, rubella, poliomyelitis, pertussis, diphtheria, *H. influenzae* type b, and tetanus are not just harmless childhood illnesses. All of them can cripple or kill.

All are preventable. In order to be completely protected against diphtheria, tetanus, and pertussis, your child needs a shot of the combination diphtheria-tetanus-pertussis (DTP) vaccine at two, four, six, and eighteen months and a booster at school time. With all but the 6-month DTP shots a drop of the oral polio vaccine (OPV) is usually given.

At 15 months your child should have a shot for measles, rubella, and mumps (MMR). This can be given in one combination shot. Children should be tested for tuberculosis in the first year of life with optional testing dependent on risk in the preschool and school-age period. *Haemophilus* b polysaccharide vaccine (HBPV) is due at 2 years. At 14 to 16 years a tetanus-diphtheria booster shot should be given.

If you don't have a pediatrician or family physician, call your local public health department. It usually has supplies of vaccine and may give shots free.

Recommended Schedule for Active Immunization of Normal Infants and Children

Recommended Age	Immunization(s)	Comments
2 mo	DTP,[1] OPV[2]	Can be initiated as early as 2 wk of age in areas of high endemicity or during epidemics
4 mo	DTP, OPV	2-mo interval desired for OPV to avoid interference from previous dose
6 mo	DTP (OPV)	OPV is optional (may be given in areas with increased risk of poliovirus exposure)
15 mo	Measles, Mumps, Rubella (MMR)[3]	MMR preferred to individual vaccines; tuberculin testing may be done (see Tuberculosis)
18 mo	DTP,[4,5] OPV[5]	
24 mo	HBPV[6]	
4–6 yr[7]	DTP, OPV	At or before school entry
14–16 yr	Td[8]	Repeat every 10 yr throughout life

[1]DTP—Diphtheria and tetanus toxoids with pertussis vaccine.
[2]OPV—Oral, poliovirus vaccine contains attenuated poliovirus types 1, 2, and 3.
[3]MMR—Live measles, mumps, and rubella viruses in a combined vaccine (see text for discussion of single vaccines versus combination).
[4]Should be given 6 to 12 months after the third dose.
[5]May be given simultaneously with MMR at 15 months of age.
[6]*Haemophilus* b polysaccharide vaccine.
[7]Up to the seventh birthday.
[8]Td—Adult tetanus toxoid (full dose) and diphtheria toxoid (reduced dose) in combination.

For all products used, consult manufacturer's package insert for instructions for storage, handling, and administration. Biologics prepared by different manufacturers may vary, and those of the same manufacturer may change from time to time. Therefore, the physician should be aware of the contents of the package insert.

Reprinted from Committee on Infectious Diseases: *Report of the Committee on Infectious Diseases*, ed 20. Elk Grove Village, IL, American Academy of Pediatrics, 1986, p 9, table 2

APPENDIX V.4

Guidelines For Letter To Parents Concerning Illness

1. Identify the cause of the infection as precisely as possible. Include the medical name of the cause of the infection and the symptoms which result (fever, cough, diarrhea, rash, etc.).
2. Indicate the length of time the parent needs to be worried about whether additional cases will occur from day care exposure.
3. Indicate how the infection is spread (cough, hand contact between stool and mouth, etc.).
   Indicate if apparently well children can carry and spread the agent.
4. State level of concern:
   a. Notify your doctor if _____develops.
   b. Call your doctor for advice.
   c. Medical advisor/health department has recommended that all children have cultures of _____ receive _____.
      This will be performed at the center or
      Please call your child's doctor to arrange that this be done.
   d. State applicability or lack of applicability of recommendations to parents, other children in the household, other close contacts (babysitter, church, school, etc.).
5. Indicate restriction on child's return to center, if any.
6. If applicable, indicate that the exposed children should stay together until control measures/incubation period has been completed.
7. Establish one or two people to answer all questions and to serve as liaisons with physicians. State how and when these people can be contacted.
8. If child becomes ill between the date of notification and the date of incubation period (state date)_____. request that the center be notified either that the illness is a possible case of _____or if the illness is due to another cause.

Adapted from: Infectious Disease Committee
Northern California Chapter
American Academy of Pediatrics
Rev. 1-11-83

APPENDIX VI.1

Sources Of Child Health And Safety Information And Materials

Federal
1. Head Start Health Service, Administration for Child, Youth and Families, P.O. Box 1182, Washington, D.C. 20013.
2. U.S. Department of Labor, Occupational Safety and Health Administration (OSHA), Washington, D.C. 20013.
3. U.S. Department of Agriculture, Food and Nutrition Information Center, National Agricultural Library Building, Room 304, Beltsville, MD 20705. 1-301-344-3719.
4. Clearinghouse on Child Abuse and Neglect Information, P.O. Box 1182, Washington, D.C. 20013. 1-202-755-0590.
5. Clearinghouse on the Handicapped, Room 338-D, Hubert H. Humphrey Building, 200 Independence Ave., S.W., Washington, D.C. 20201. 1-202-245-1961.
6. Clearinghouse on Sudden Infant Death Syndrome (SIDS), 1555 Wilson Blvd., Suite 600, Rosslyn, VA 22209-2461. 1-703-522-0870.
7. National Information Center for Handicapped Children and Youth, 1555 Wilson Blvd., Rosslyn, VA 22209. 1-703-522-0870.
8. National Institute of Mental Health (NIMH), 5600 Fishers Lane, Rockville, MD 20857.
9. National Institute of Child Health and Human Development, Office of Research Reporting, 9600 Rockville Pike, Room 2A-32, Bethesda, MD 20205. 1-301-496-5133.
10. For anything developed by or procured through the Division of Maternal and Child Health, write to: Health Clearinghouse, 8201 Greensboro Drive, Suite 600, McLean, VA 22102.
11. Superintendent of Documents, Government Printing Office, Washington, D.C. 20402.
12. United States Consumer Product Safety Commission, (USCPSC), Room 336B, 5401 Westband Ave., Bethesda, MD 20207. 1-800-638-2772.

National (private)

1. American Academy of Pediatrics, Division of Health Education, 141 Northwest Point Blvd., P.O. Box 927, Elk Grove Village, IL 60009. 1-800-433-0797. Resources: The Injury Prevention Program (TIPP): parent questionnaires and handouts with instructions for preventing injuries to children, child passenger safety pamphlets, the newsletter *Safe Ride News*, and the handbook Injury Prevention in Children and Youth (in press).
2. National Child Passenger Safety Association. Contact: Elaine Weinstein, 1705 DeSales Street, N.W., Suite 300, Washington, D.C. 20036. 1-202-429-0515. Resources: pamphlet, quarterly newsletter, national networking child safety advocates, general information clearinghouse on child passenger safety.
3. Physicians for Automotive Safety. Contact: Annemarie Shelners, P.O. Box 430, Armonk, NY 10504. 1-914-173-6446. Resources: pamphlets, parent education films, slides, quarterly newsletter.
4. National Fire Protection Association, Batterymarch Park, Quincy, MA 02269. 1-800-344-3555.
5. American Society for Testing and Materials, 1916 Race Street, Philadelphia, PA 19103.
6. National Safety Council, 444 N. Michigan Ave., Chicago, Ill. 1-312-527-4800.
7. National Association for the Education of Young Children, 1834 Connecticut Ave., N.W., Washington, D.C. 20009. 1-800-424-2460.
8. Child Care Information Exchange, P.O. Box 2890, Redmond, WA 98073. 1-206-882-1066.
9. American Red Cross National Headquarters, Health Services, 17th & D Street, N.W., Washington, D.C. 20006.
10. American Home Economics Association, 2010 Massachusetts Ave., N.W., Washington, D.C. 20036.
11. March of Dimes, Supply Division, 1275 Mamaroneck Ave., White Plains, NY 10605.
12. Society for Nutrition Education, 1736 Franklin Street, Oakland, CA 94612.
13. Metropolitan Life Insurance Company, Health and Welfare Film Library, c/o Association Films, Inc., 600 Aronid Ave., Ridgefreed, NJ 07657. 1-201-943-8200. Or One Madison Ave., New York, NY 10010. 1-212-578-5015.

14. Safety Now Company, Inc., P.O. Box 567, Jenkintown, PA 19046.
15. Preschool Enrichment Team, Inc., c/o Patricia Wise, R.N., 276 High St., Holyoke, MA 01040. A poster source for hand washing techniques and day care health training.
16. Child Welfare League of America, Inc., 67 Irving Place, New York, NY 10003.

State and Local (public)

1. "Safe Schools," a guide to creating safe environments for preschoolers. (A how-to manual for teachers.) Department of Public Health, Division of Family Health Services, 150 Tremont St., Boston, MA 02111.
2. Cooperative Extension Service, located in different offices in each state.
3. Police departments, state and local.
4. Fire departments, local.
5. State and local injury prevention projects. These may be in local health departments, or in local hospitals, and in state health offices.
6. Child protective services. These may be located in different offices within the state and local welfare or human service agencies.
7. State and local health departments and within them their offices for environmental protection, maternal and child health, and health education.

State and local (private)

1. State and local medical societies.
2. State and local dental societies.
3. Association for the Blind, state and local chapters.
4. Lung Association, state and local chapters.
5. American Automobile Association, local office.

APPENDIX VI.2

SITE SAFETY CHECKLIST

Date Inspection Was Made _____

Name of Person Performing Inspection _____

Rooms and Units	Satisfactory		Corrections Needed	Date Corrections Made
Floors are smooth, clean and have a nonskid surface.	OK	Not OK		
Medicines, cleaning agents and tools are inaccessible to children. There are no aerosols in the room. Art supplies are nontoxic.	OK	Not OK		
First aid kit is present and adequately supplied. No medicines are unlocked.	OK	Not OK		
Walls, ceiling clean and in repair. No peeling paint, damaged plaster. Less than 20% of wall surface is covered by hangings.	OK	Not OK		
Children are never unattended, always supervised by enough staff to evacuate.	OK	Not OK		
Lighting and electricity: brightness is OK, outlets are covered, no dangling or covered extension cords.	OK	Not OK		

Rooms and Units	Satisfactory		Corrections Needed	Date Corrections Made
No free standing space heater.	OK	Not OK		
Heating and ventilation systems are working OK. Pipes and radiators are inaccessible or covered to prevent body contact if 110°F or above.	OK	Not OK		
Humidity level is comfortable.	OK	Not OK		
Hand washing facility: hot water temperature should not exceed 110°F (43°C), facility is easily accessible, soap and towel supplies are adequate.	OK	Not OK		
No disease-bearing animals, vermin or poisonous plants (no turtles, hamsters or harmful pets).	OK	Not OK		
Trash storage is covered. Sanitation adequate especially in food service areas, cots or mats, dust traps.	OK	Not OK		
Exits are clearly marked and unobstructed. Easy access to emergency phone. Emergency contact information is current.	OK	Not OK		
Locked doors to closed spaces can be opened by an adult.	OK	Not OK		
No smoking in child care area.	OK	Not OK		

Rooms and Units	Satisfactory		Corrections Needed	Date Corrections Made
No precariously placed small or sharp or otherwise hazardous objects. Plastic bags are safely used.	OK	Not OK		
Rest equipment is labeled. Linens, mats, cribs, cots, and blankets appear clean.	OK	Not OK		
Toys and furnishings are in repair and free of pinch or crush points.	OK	Not OK		
Decor is pleasant, nonflammable materials are used.	OK	Not OK		
Windows securely screened and opening limited to 6 inches.	OK	Not OK		
Fans in use have covers or guards with openings smaller than one half inch.	OK	Not OK		
Infant Toddler Programs Toys are lead-free. Mouthed toys are sanitized between different children's use.	OK	Not OK		
High chairs have wide base and safety strap.	OK	Not OK		
Diaper changing area clean, adequately supplied with changing pads and disposable sheeting. Sanitized after each use.	OK	Not OK		
Soiled diapers disposed of in securely tied plastic bag.	OK	Not OK		
No bottles in crib or infants lying down drinking.	OK	Not OK		

Rooms and Units	Satisfactory		Corrections Needed	Date Corrections Made
No toddlers walking around with bottles.	OK	Not OK		
Hand washing for child and caregivers practiced after each diaper change.	OK	Not OK		

Hallways and Stairs	Satisfactory		Corrections Needed	Date Corrections Made
Smoke detectors are OK	OK	Not OK		
Exits are neither obstructed nor cluttered. Clear exit routes are marked. Alarm system is working. Fire extinguishers OK. Emergency lighting is OK.	OK	Not OK		
Monitoring for entrance of strangers is consistently done. Emergency phone numbers (police, fire, rescue, poison control) are posted by phone.	OK	Not OK		
Doors open in direction of exit travel.	OK	Not OK		
Doors are operational with panic hardware on emergency exits. Windows are screened.	OK	Not OK		
Floors are smooth, clean and have a nonskid surface. Rugs are attached.	OK	Not OK		
Walls are painted with lead free paint. Plaster is intact. There are no loose nails or other hazards.	OK	Not OK		

Hallways and Stairs	Satisfactory		Corrections Needed	Date Corrections Made
There are no disease bearing animals, vermin or poisonous plants (no turtles, hamsters or harmful pets).	OK	Not OK		
Heating and ventilation are working OK. Pipes and radiators are inaccessible or covered to prevent body contact. Humidity level is comfortable.	OK	Not OK		
Lighting electricity: Brightness OK. Outlets are covered. There are no dangling or covered extension cords.	OK	Not OK		
Right hand descending railing secured at child height.	OK	Not OK		
Stairs and stairways free of stored items. Stairways well lit by artificial or natural light.	OK	Not OK		
Safeguards to prevent children from entering unsupervised or hazardous areas.	OK	Not OK		
Clear glass panels used in traffic areas are safety glass or equivalent and are clearly marked to avoid accidental impact.	OK	Not OK		
Fans in use have covers or guards with openings smaller than one half inch.	OK	Not OK		

Kitchen and Storage Areas	Satisfactory		Corrections Needed	Date Corrections Made
Plumbing and water temperature: at least 170°F water or sanitizing agent is used for sanitization. Plumbing is working properly.	OK	Not OK		
Trash storage covered and litter minimum. Trash kept away from potential food storage and preparation areas. No storage near furnace or hot water heaters.	OK	Not OK		
Heating and ventilation systems are working OK. Pipes and radiators are inaccessible or covered to prevent body contact. Humidity level is comfortable.	OK	Not OK		
No animals or vermin are present. Insects are controlled by screens. No pesticides are used on food, food preparation or storage surfaces.	OK	Not OK		
No pest strips or pesticides used where possible contact with food can occur.	OK	Not OK		
Cleaning agents and tools and utensils including matches are stored away from food storage and used safely. Toxic materials are in original containers separately stored away from food.	OK	Not OK		

Kitchen and Storage Areas	Satisfactory		Corrections Needed	Date Corrections Made
Lighting and electricity: Brightness is OK, outlets are covered, there are no dangling or covered extension cords. Fire extinguishers in safe working order.	OK	Not OK		
Food Storage: Inventory and dated rotation methods are used. Refrigerator temperatures less than 45°F. Frozen foods are stored at 0°F or below. Handled leftovers are discarded.	OK	Not OK		
Food is stored on shelves; containers are labeled; made of insect resistant metal or plastic (not plastic bags).	OK	Not OK		
First aid kit is available and adequately stocked.	OK	Not OK		
Fire extinguisher is charged. Staff know how to use it.	OK	Not OK		
Personnel are healthy and perform appropriate, frequent hand washing, use hair restraints, wear clean clothing. No smoking allowed in food preparation area.	OK	Not OK		
Sanitation: Surfaces are clean, free of cracks or crevices. Wood cutting boards are not used.	OK	Not OK		
Eating utensils are free of cracks and chips.	OK	Not OK		

Kitchen and Storage Areas	Satisfactory		Corrections Needed	Date Corrections Made
Pot handles on stove are turned inward where they cannot be knocked over and contents spilled.	OK	Not OK		

Outdoors	Satisfactory		Corrections Needed	Date Corrections Made
Free of litter and sharp objects.	OK	Not OK		
Play equipment is smooth, well anchored and free of rust, splinters or sharp corners. No exposed uncapped screws or bolts. Size appropriate to child users. Bars stay in place when grasped. Maximum height, 6 feet. Safe way out on all climbers.	OK	Not OK		
No "S" hooks or other open hooks. Swing seats are light-weight, flexible and noncutting. Equipment is placed in safe location (away from where other children would play).	OK	Not OK		
Slides have horizontal steps and good tread. Rim on slide to prevent falls, flat bottom to slow down. Metal beds are shaded from the sun. Steps 7 inches apart, flat (not tubular).	OK	Not OK		

Outdoors	Satisfactory		Corrections Needed	Date Corrections Made
Are sandboxes covered when not in use? Places for adults to sit where needed to supervise?	OK	Not OK		
Rings do not permit entry of child's head or they are large enough for whole body.	OK	Not OK		
No pinch or crush points on equipment.	OK	Not OK		
Fences or natural barriers prohibit access to hazardous areas and keep animals out.	OK	Not OK		
No stagnant pools of water.	OK	Not OK		
Playground surface is nonabrasive, and impact-absorbing (shredded tires, wood chips), free of litter and concealed debris; no animal excrement.	OK	Not OK		
Poisonous plants and stinging insect nests removed.	OK	Not OK		
Street traffic controlled. Pick-up and drop-off procedures are safe.	OK	Not OK		
Vehicles				
School bus signs are in place.	OK	Not OK		
Vehicles are mechanically in order.	OK	Not OK		
Safety restraints are adequate in number and type and are used.	OK	Not OK		

Outdoors	Satisfactory		Corrections Needed	Date Corrections Made
Safety locks or child door-opening restraints present.	OK	Not OK		
Driver training for school bus safety is up-to-date.	OK	Not OK		
Attendants present as required.	OK	Not OK		
First aid kit is adequately stocked.	OK	Not OK		
Current emegency contact and medical information is in vehicle when in use.	OK	Not OK		
Trips are planned with emergency management and health facilities identified beforehand.	OK	Not OK		
Children have identification including their name, and emergency contacts.	OK	Not OK		
Bathroom and Laundry Room	Satisfactory		Corrections Needed	Date Corrections Made
Hand washing facility: hot water temperature is less than 120°F, facility is easily accessible, soap and towel supplies are adequate.	OK	Not OK		
Covered lids on trash in adults' bathroom. Trash storage and litter is adequately controlled.	OK	Not OK		
Cleaning agents are inaccessible to children. No other toxic products stored in area.	OK	Not OK		

Bathroom and Laundry Room	Satisfactory		Corrections Needed	Date Corrections Made
Windows, doors, ceilings, walls are clean and well maintained. Floors are not slippery.	OK	Not OK		
Temperature and ventilation are adequately and safely maintained.	OK	Not OK		
Toilets and sinks are age-appropriate size or adapted. Step stools are provided where appropriate. No potty chairs.	OK	Not OK		
There is no electrical equipment near water.	OK	Not OK		
Exits are clearly marked.	OK	Not OK		
Animals and vermin are controlled.	OK	Not OK		
Towels, toilet tissues and soap (liquid, not bar) are available.	OK	Not OK		
Other	OK	Not OK		

From: Aronson, S., Nelson, H.
Health Power
Westinghouse Health Systems, Inc.
1976
Updated by S. Aronson 12/85

APPENDIX VI.3

Occupational Safety And Health Administration (OSHA)

Consultation Service Project Directory

A directory of offices providing advice on safety to individuals responsible for programs at nongovernment work sites.

STATE	TELEPHONE
Alabama	(205) 348-7136
Alaska	(907) 276-5013
Arizona	(602) 255-5795
Arkansas	(501) 375-8442
California	(415) 557-2870
Colorado	(303) 491-6151
Connecticut	(203) 566-4550
Delaware	(302) 571-3908
District of Columbia	(202) 576-6651
Florida	(904) 488-3044
Georgia	(404) 894-3806
Guam	9-011 (671) 477-9821
Hawaii	(808) 548-2511
Idaho	(208) 385-3929
Illinois	(800) 972-4140/4216 (Toll-free in State) (312) 793-3270
Indiana	(317) 232-2688
Iowa	(515) 281-5352
Kansas	(913) 296-4386
Kentucky	(502) 564-6895
Louisiana	No Services Available
Maine	(207) 289-2591
Maryland	(301) 659-4218
Massachusetts	(617) 727-3463
Michigan	(517) 373-1410 (H) (517) 322-1809 (S)

STATE	TELEPHONE
Minnesota	(612) 297-1953 (S)
	(612) 623-5100 (H)
Mississippi	(601) 982-6315
Missouri	(314) 751-3403
Montana	(406) 444-6401
Navajo Nation	(602) 871-6335
Nebraska	(402) 471-2239
Nevada	(702) 885-5240
New Hampshire	(603) 271-3170
New Jersey	(609) 984-3507
New Mexico	(505) 827-8949
New York	(212) 488-7746/7
North Carolina	(919) 733-4880
North Dakota	(701) 224-2366
Ohio	(800) 282-1425
	(Toll-free in State)
	(614) 466-7485
Oklahoma	(405) 521-2461
Oregon	(503) 378-3273
Pennsylvania	(800) 382-1241
	(Toll-free in State)
	(412) 357-3019
Puerto Rico	(809) 754-2134/2171
Rhode Island	(401) 277-2438
South Carolina	(803) 758-8921
South Dakota	(605) 688-4101
Tennessee	(615) 741-2793
Texas	(512) 458-7287
Utah	(801) 530-6868
Vermont	(802) 828-2765
Virginia	(804) 786-5875 (S)
	(804) 786-6285 (H)
Virgin Islands	(809) 772-1315
Washington	(206) 753-6500
West Virginia	(304) 348-7890
Wisconsin	(608) 266-0417 (H)
	(414) 521-5063 (S)
Wyoming	(307) 777-7786

APPENDIX VI.4

Fourteen Ways To Avoid Plant Poisoning

1. Become familiar with the dangerous plants in your area, yard, and home. Know them by sight and name.
2. Do not eat wild plants, including mushrooms, unless *positive* of identification.
3. Keep plants, seeds, fruits, and bulbs away from infants.
4. Teach children at an early age to keep unknown plants and plant parts out of their mouths. Make them aware of the potential danger of poisonous plants.
5. Teach children to recognize poison ivy or other causes of dermatitis in your area.
6. Be certain you know the plants used by children as playthings (seeds or fruits, stems, etc.) or as skewers for meat or marshmallows.
7. Do not allow children to suck nectar from flowers or make "tea" from leaves.
8. Know the plant before eating its fruits.
9. Do not rely on pets, birds, or squirrels to indicate nonpoisonous plants.
10. Avoid smoke from burning plants, unless you know exactly what they are.
11. Remember, heating and cooking do not always destroy the toxic substance.
12. Store labeled bulbs and seeds safely away from children and pets.
13. Do not make homemade medicines from native or cultivated plants.
14. Remember, there are no safe "tests" or "rules of thumb" for distinguishing edible from poisonous plants.

Source: *Human Poisoning from Native and Cultivated Plants*, second edition, James W. Hardin and Jay M. Arena, M.D., Duke University Press, Durham, North Carolina, 1974.

POISONOUS PLANTS

Children are often attracted to the colorful berries, flowers, fruits and leaves of plants. But over 700 plants in the U.S.

and Canada have been identified as poisonous. These can be found anywhere—in your neighbor's or your own house, in florist shops and grocery stores, in yards, in the woods and on playgrounds.

Plants are a common cause of poisoning to preschoolers. Most of these poisonings can be prevented, so it's important for parents, grandparents, babysitters and day care workers to know if poisonous plants are near children.

If eaten, some plant parts can cause a skin rash or stomach upset; others can even cause death. Here is a partial list of indoor and outdoor plants that are very dangerous—children have died from eating these.

Autumn crocus	Lantana
Azalea	Laurel
Baneberry	Lily-of-the-valley
Belladonna	Lupine
Black cherry	Mistletoe
Black locust	Monkshood
Black snakeroot	Moonseed
Buckeye	Mountain laurel
Caladium	Mushrooms
Caper spurge	Nightshade
Castor bean	Oleander
Cherry	Poison hemlock
Chinaberry	Pokeweed
Daffodil bulbs	Privet
Daphne	Rhododendron
Delphinium	Rhubarb leaves
Dieffenbacchia	Rosary pea
Dumbcane	Rubber vine
Duranta	Sandbox tree
False hellebore	Tansy
Foxglove	Thorn apple
Golden chain	Tobacco
Hyacinth	Tung oil tree
Hydrangea	Water hemlock
Jequirity bean	White snakeroot
Jessamine	Yellow jessamine
Jimsonweed	Yellow oleander
Larkspur	Yew

There is no rule of thumb to help you tell a poisonous plant from a safe one. You can get help in identifying plants from library books, garden and florist shops.

If you think your child may have swallowed any part of a poisonous plant, first remove any remaining pieces from the child's mouth. Then bring a piece of the plant to the phone and call the local poison control center. Refer to Poison under Emergency numbers in your local telephone book.

SAFE HOUSEPLANTS

A sure way to prevent these poisonings inside the home is by substituting safe plants for poisonous ones. Here is a list of some common indoor plants that are safe for growing around young children.

COMMON NAME	BOTANICAL NAME
African violet	Saintpaulia ionantha
Aluminum plant	Pilea cadierei
Begonia	Begonia semperflorens
Boston fern	Nephrolepis exaltata
Coleus	Coleus blumei
Dracaena	Dracaena fragrans
Hens-and-chickens	Sempervivum tectorum
Jade plant	Crassula argentea
Mother-in-law's tongue	Sansevieria trifasciata
Peperomia	Peperomia obtusifolia
Prayer plant	Maranta leuconeura
Rubber plant	Ficus elastica
Sensitive plant	Mimosa pudica
Spider plant	Shlorophytum comosum
Swedish ivy	Plectranthus australis
Wandering Jew	Tradescantia fluminensis
Wax plant	Hoya carnosa
Weeping fig	Ficus benjamina

Adapted from:
  SCIPP
  Statewide Comprehensive Injury Prevention Program
  Massachusetts Department of Public Health
  Division of Family Health Services
  150 Tremont Street, 3rd Floor
  Boston, MA 02111
  (617) 727-1246

APPENDIX VI.5

Unsafe Art Supplies

AVOID powdered clay. It contains silica, which is easily inhaled and harmful to the lungs.
USE wet clay which can't be inhaled.

AVOID glazes that contain lead.
USE poster paints.

AVOID paints that require solvents such as turpentine to clean brushes.
USE water-based paints.

AVOID cold-water or commercial dyes that contain chemical additives.
USE natural dyes, such as vegetables, onion skins, etc.

AVOID permanent markers, which may contain toxic solvents.
USE water-based markers.

AVOID instant papier mache, which may contain lead or asbestos.
USE black-and-white newspaper and library paste or liquid starch.

AVOID epoxy, instant glues, or other solvent-based glues.
USE water-based white glue or library paste.

AVOID powdered tempera paints.
USE liquid paint or any nontoxic paint.

For more information contact:
Art Hazards Information Center
5 Beekman Street
New York City, NY 10038

APPENDIX VI.6

First Aid Instructions

The following are safe first aid measures for various types of poisoning:

SWALLOWED POISONS—This is an emergency—any nonfood substance is a potential poison.

Call physician, poison control center, or hospital emergency department promptly for advice.

Do not make the patient vomit if:

- Patient is unconscious or drowsy
- Patient is convulsing or having tremors (or "twitching" of the arms and/or legs or having uncontrolled body movements)
- Patient swallowed a strong corrosive (such as drain cleaner, oven cleaner, toilet bowl cleaner, strong acids)
- Patient swallowed furniture polish, kerosene, gasoline, or other petroleum products (except after specific medical advice)

Directions for making a patient vomit:

- Use syrup of Ipecac. (Do not give salt water.)
- For children under 12 months of age, obtain medical advice.
- For children one to ten years of age, give 3 teaspoons (one tablespoon or .5 oz) syrup of Ipecac followed by 4 to 8 oz of water. If no vomiting occurs in 20 minutes, repeat dose once only.
- For children over ten years of age, give 2 tablespoons (1 oz) Ipecac syrup followed by 4 to 8 oz water.

If instructed, drive carefully to medical facility. Take pan to collect vomitus. Bring package or container with intact label of material ingested or whatever left over material there is.

FUMES OR GASES—Fuel gases, auto exhaust, dense smoke from fires or fumes from poisonous chemicals.

• Get victim into fresh air.
• Loosen clothing.
• If victim is not breathing, start artificial respiration promptly. Do not stop until patient is breathing well, or help arrives.
• Have *someone else* call a physician, poison control center, hospital, or rescue unit.
• Transport victim to a medical facility promptly.

EYE

• Holding lids open, flush out eye immediately with water,
• Remove contact lenses if worn,
• Irrigate eye for 15 minutes with a gentle continuous stream of water from a pitcher.
• Never permit eye to be rubbed or use eye drops.
• Call physician, poison control center, or emergency department for further advice.

SKIN—Acids, lye, other caustics, pesticides, etc.

• Brush off dry material gently. Then immediately wash off skin with a large amount of water; use soap if available.
• Remove any contaminated clothing.
• Call physician, poison control center, or emergency department for further advice.

BITES AND STINGS

SNAKE

Non-Poisonous
- Treat as a puncture wound. Consult physician.
  Poisonous
- Put patient and injured part at rest. Keep quiet.
- Do not apply ice. May use cool compress for pain.
- Immediate suction without incision may be beneficial.
- Apply loose (allow two fingers under) constricting band above the bite (not around fingers or toes) if cannot get to medical help in one hour.
- Transport victim promptly to a medical facility.

INSECTS—Spiders, scorpions, or unusual reaction to other stinging insects such as bees, wasps, hornets, etc.

- Remove stinger if present with a scraping motion of a plastic card or fingernail to reduce injection of more toxin. Do not pull out.
- Use cold compresses on bite area to relieve pain.
- If victim stops breathing, use artificial respiration and have someone call rescue unit and physician for further instructions.
- If any reactions such as hives, generalized rash, pallor, weakness, nausea, vomiting, "tightness" in chest, nose, or throat, or collapse occurs, get patient to physician or emergency department immediately.
- For scorpion sting, get immediate medical advice.
- For spider bites, obtain medical advice. (Save live specimen if safe and possible.)

TICKS

- Always thoroughly inspect child after time in woods or brush. Ticks carry many serious diseases and must be com-

pletely removed.
- Use tweezers or protected fingers placed close to the head to pull tick away from point of attachment.
- If head breaks off, victim should be taken without delay for medical removal.

ANIMAL—Bat, racoon, skunk, and fox bites, as well as unprovoked bites from cats and dogs, may be from a rabid animal.

- Call physician or medical facility.
- Wash wound gently but thoroughly with soap and water for 15 minutes.

POISONOUS MARINE ANIMALS—Stingray, lionfish, catfish, and stonefish stings

- Put victim at rest and submerge sting area in hot water.
- Call physician or medical facility.

OTHER MARINE STINGS

- Flush with water, remove any clinging material.
- Apply cold compress to relieve pain.
- Call physician or medical facility.

SKIN WOUNDS—Protection against tetanus should be considered in all burns and whenever the skin is broken.

BRUISES

Rest injured part. Apply cold compress for half hour (no ice next to skin). If skin is broken, treat as a cut. For wringer injuries and bicycle spoke injuries, always consult physician without delay.

SCRAPES

Use wet gauze or cotton to sponge off gently with clean water and soap. Apply sterile dressing, preferably nonadhesive or "film" type (Telfapad).

CUTS

Small
   Wash with clean water and soap. Hold under running water. Apply sterile gauze dressing.

Large
   Apply dressing. Press firmly and elevate to stop bleeding— use tourniquet only if necessary to control bleeding. Bandage. Secure medical care. Do not use iodine or other antiseptics without medical advice.

PUNCTURE WOUNDS

   Consult physician.

SLIVERS

   Wash with clean water and soap. Remove with tweezers or forceps. Wash again. If not easily removed, consult physician.

BITES AND STINGS

   See Poisoning.

BURNS AND SCALDS—Protection against tetanus should be considered in all burns and whenever the skin is broken.

BURNS OF LIMITED EXTENT

If caused by heat:
- Immerse extremity burns in cool water or apply cool (50° to 60°F) compresses to burns of the trunk or face for pain relief.
- Do not break blisters.
- Nonadhesive material such as household aluminum foil makes an excellent emergency covering.
- Burns of any size of the face, hands, feet, or genitalia should be seen immediately by a physician.

EXTENSIVE BURNS

- Keep patient in a flat position.
- Remove nonadherent clothing from burn area—if not easily removed, leave alone.
- Apply cool wet compresses to injured area (not more than 25% of the body at one time).
- Keep patient warm.
- Get patient to hospital or physician at once.
- Do not use ointments, greases, powder, etc.

ELECTRIC BURNS

- Disconnect power source if possible, or pull victim away from source using wood or cloth.
- Do not use bare hands.
- Electric burns may require "CPR" (Cardio Pulmonary Resuscitation).
- All electric burns must be evaluated by a physician.

SUNBURN

Children under one year of age may suffer serious injury and should be examined by a physician.

FRACTURES

Any deformity of injured part usually means a fracture. Do not move person without splinting. Suspected neck or back injury should only be moved with medical assistance to avoid causing paralysis.

SPRAINS

Elevate injured part and apply only *cold* compresses. If marked pain or swelling present, seek medical advice.

TEETH

KNOCKED-OUT TOOTH

• If the tooth is dirty, rinse it gently in running water. Do not scrub it.
• Gently insert and hold the tooth in its socket. If this is not possible, place the tooth in a container of milk or cool water.
• Go immediately to your dentist (within 30 minutes, if possible). Don't forget to bring the tooth.

BROKEN TOOTH

• Gently clean dirt or debris from the injured area with warm water.
• Place cold compresses on the face in the area of the injured tooth to minimize swelling.
• Go to the dentist immediately.

EYES

Do not apply pressure to eye or instill medications without physician's advice.

- Attempt removal of foreign body by gentle use of moist cotton swab; if not immediately successful, obtain medical assistance. Pain in eye from foreign bodies, scrapes, scratches, cuts, etc. can be alleviated by bandaging the lids shut until doctor's aid can be obtained.
- For chemicals splashed in eyes, flush immediately with plain water and continue for 15 minutes. Do not use drops or ointments. Call physician or poison control center.
- If eye perforated by missile or sharp object, do not apply pressure to lids and avoid straining. Consult ophthalmologist immediately.
- If eye received blunt trauma, consult physician if in doubt, especially if there is blurring or double vision, flashing lights or floating specks.

NOSEBLEEDS

In sitting position, squeeze outside of nostrils between thumb and index finger for five to ten minutes. If bleeding persists, call your physician.

FAINTING

Keep in flat position. Loosen clothing around neck. Turn head to side. Keep patient warm. Keep mouth clear. Give nothing to swallow. Obtain medical aid.

HEAD INJURIES

Complete rest. Consult physician. Obtain additional consultation if:
- There is a loss of consciousness at any time thereafter.
- You are unable to arouse the child from sleep. (You may allow the child to sleep after the injury but check frequently to see whether the child can be aroused. Check at least every one to two hours during the day, and two to three times during the night.)
- There is persistent vomiting.

- Inability to move a limb.
- Oozing of blood or watery fluid from the ears or nose.
- Persistent headache lasting over one hour. The headache will be severe enough to interfere with activity and normal sleep.
- Persistent dizziness for one hour after the injury.
- Unequal pupils.
- Pale color that does not return to normal in a short time.

CONVULSIONS

Seek medical advice. Lay on side with head lower than hips. Put nothing in mouth. Sponge with cool water if fever present.

CHOKING

If an infant under one year of age chokes and is unable to breathe he is placed face down over the rescuer's arm with head lower than the trunk. The rescuer rests his forearm on his thigh. Four measured blows are rapidly delivered with the heel of the hand between the infant's shoulder blades. (A) If breathing is not started, the infant is rolled over and four rapid compressions of the chest are performed as for CPR (see below).
A choking child over one year of age should be placed on his back with the rescuer kneeling next to him and placing the heel of one hand on the child's abdomen in the midline between umbilicus and rib cage. A series of six to ten abdominal thrusts—Heimlich maneuver—(rapid inward and upward thrusts) should be applied until the foreign body 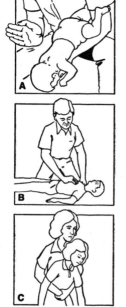 is expelled. (B) The older, larger child can be treated in a sitting, standing or recumbent position using two hands for the thrusts. (C)

If breathing is not started, open mouth with thumb over tongue and fingers wrapped around lower jaw. If a foreign body is seen it may be removed with a finger sweep.

Rapid transport to a medical facility is urgent if these emergency first aid measures fail.

CARDIOPULMONARY RESUSCITATION (CPR)

To be used in situations such as drownings, electric shock, and smoke inhalation. Technique of pulmonary support
- Clear the throat (see section on choking) and wipe out any fluid, vomitus, mucous, or foreign body.
- Place victim on back.
- Straighten neck (unless neck injury suspected) and lift jaw.
- Blow gently into infant's nose and mouth and into larger child's mouth with nostrils pinched closed.
- Breathe at 20 breaths/min for infants and 15 breaths/min for children, using only enough air to move chest up and down.

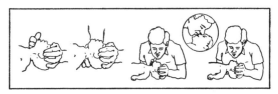

Technique of cardiac support (if no pulse or heart beat)
- Place victim on firm surface.
- In the infant, using three fingers depress breastbone ½-1″ at level of nipples. Compress at 100 times/minute.
- In the child, depress lower ⅓ of breastbone with finger or heel of hand at 80 compressions/minute. There should be five compressions to one respiration.
- Learn and practice CPR.

From:
American Academy of Pediatrics
Committee on Accident and Poison Prevention
©1986

APPENDIX VI.7

Injury Report Form

Name of Child _____ Birth Date _____

Parent Name _____

Address _____ Phone Number _____

Usual Source of Health Care _____

Date of Injury _____Time _____ Age ____ Sex ____

Type of Injury (circle) Bite, Broken Bone, Bruise, Burn, Choking, Cut, Eye Injury, Foreign Body, Head Injury, Poisoning,
   Scrape, Sliver, Sprain, Sting, Other _____

Location Where Injury Occurred _____
   e.g., child care room, bathroom, hall, playground, large
   muscle room, bus, car, walk

Type of Equipment Involved _____

How Injury Happened (who, what, where, how, when) ____

_____

_____

_____

_____

Type of Treatment Required _____
   e.g., first aid only in day care, visit to doctor's office or
   clinic, emergency room, hospitalized/sutures, cast, bandage,
   medication given

Witnesses of Injury Incident _____

Signatures of Witnesses _____

Name of Medical Professional Consulted _____

   Date _____ Time _____ Advice _____

_____

Retrospectively, what would have prevented this injury?

_____

_____

_____

_____

APPENDIX VII.1

Planning And Evaluation Form For Training In Day Care

AGENDA ITEM	BEHAVIORAL OBJECTIVES	CONCEPTS	METHODS	TIME	MATERIALS, EQUIPMENT	EVALUATION

Prepared by Susan S. Aronson, M.D.

APPENDIX VII.2

Medical Terms For The Child Day Care Professional

1. *Antibody*: Antibodies are substances produced in the body in response to a specific antigen. Antibodies help protect against antigens that gain entrance into body tissues.
2. *Antigen*: A substance foreign to the body (usually a protein, sometimes a carbohydrate) that causes the production of an antibody by the immune system.
3. *Asymptomatic*: Without symptoms. A child may, for instance, be an asymptomatic carrier of the organism that can cause strep throat (group A beta hemolytic streptococci).
4. *Bacteria*: Organisms with a cell wall. These organisms are much larger than viruses and can usually be effectively treated with antibiotics.
5. *Bacteriostatic*: A substance which inhibits growth of bacteria.
6. *Bilirubin*: A substance which is made in the liver. This substance increases in liver disease such as hepatitis and can cause yellowing of the skin or eyes (yellowing of parts of the body is called "jaundice").
7. *Bronchitis*: Inflammation of the air passage tubes leading into the lungs.
8. *Cellulitis*: A spreading infection involving the skin and area below the skin. This infection usually results from infection by specific bacteria (e.g., *Streptococcus*, *Staphylococcus*, and *Haemophilus influenzae*).
9. *Chart*: A record of information in text or tables. For example, when a child visits the physician, information is placed on the patient's chart.
10. *Chickenpox*: A highly infectious disease caused by the virus Varicella-zoster. The incubation period after exposure ranges from 10 to 21 days. The disease includes fever, muscle aches, and a rash. The rash appears usually as small blisters (vesicles). Children can spread disease 1 to 2 days before the rash appears and 5 to 6 days after the first blisters appear.

11. *Carrier*: A child who is infected with a specific organism but has no symptoms of disease. For example, some children may be asymptomatic carriers of the organism *Haemophilus influenzae* or *Streptococcus pyogenes* (which causes "strep" throat).
12. *Communicable period*: The period of time when a child is capable of spreading infection to another child. In chickenpox, this period is 1 to 2 days before the onset of rash and 5 to 6 days after the first group of blisters has appeared. A list of the communicable periods for common diseases of childhood is given at the end of this glossary.
13. *Conjunctivitis*: Inflammation of the delicate tissue which lines the eyelids and covers the eyeball.
14. *Coryza*: Discharge from the nose (runny nose). Occurs with the common cold.
15. *Croup*: Spasm of the air passage causing noisy and sometimes difficult breathing. Croup can be caused by a number of different bacteria and viruses.
16. *Defervescence*: Decline in fever.
17. *Diarrhea*: An increase in amount and change in quality (too loose or watery) of stool. The following organisms can cause diarrhea: rotavirus, Norwalk virus, *Salmonella, Giardia, Shigella, Campylobacter, Clostridium difficile, E. coli.*
18. *Dyspnea*: Difficulty in breathing or shortness of breath. For example, a dyspnea may occur in a child with pneumonia.
19. *Emesis*: The act of vomiting.
20. *Encephalitis*: Inflammation of the brain which can be caused by a number of viruses including those that cause mumps, measles, and chickenpox.
21. *Epiglottis*: This is the tissue lid that covers the opening to the air passage when food is being swallowed. When this organ becomes swollen and inflamed (called epiglottitis), it can interfere with breathing.
22. *Fomite*: An inanimate object or material. If certain disease-producing agents are located on fomites, then the fomites can serve as a means for spreading those agents.
23. *Erythema*: Redness of the skin. Often used as an adjective, for example, an erythematous lesion.
24. *Giardia*: *Giardia lamblia* is the name of a protozoan that can cause infections with diarrhea in children in day care settings. It can cause diarrhea, anorexia (lack of

desire to eat), and nausea. Many children may be asymptomatic.

25. *Haemophilus influenzae*: This bacterial organism may cause meningitis, cellulitis, pneumonia, otitis media, epiglottitis, or conjunctivitis.

26. *Hepatitis*: This term refers to inflammation of the liver. There are three common types of hepatitis: type A, type B, and non-A, non-B. Hepatitis type A is transmitted by the fecal-oral route and is often asymptomatic in children. It has been documented as a frequent cause of hepatitis in day care (see #32 in this glossary). Hepatitis type B, and non-A, non-B have not been identified as significant problems in day care.

27. *Host*: A person or animal that supports an infectious agent.

28. *Hypothesis*: A proposed explanation for observations; can be tested by appropriate studies.

29. *Icterus*: Another word for jaundice, a yellowing of the skin tissue or the whites of the eyes. For example, a physician may say a child has "icteric" eyes.

30. *Immunity*: This term refers to the protection from or resistance to infection that a person may acquire. A child acquires immunity to measles, mumps, rubella, and pertussis after immunization. Newborn children initially have the same immune status as their mothers. This usually wanes during the first six months of life.

31. *Immunization*: This is the process of giving active immunity to children (i.e., baby shots). The immunizing agent is usually an inactivated or killed agent, or may be an attenuated live organism such as measles or polio vaccine. The currently recommended schedule for active immunization of healthy infants and children is listed below:

Recommended Age	Immunization
2 months	DTP, OPV
4 months	DTP, OPV
6 months	DTP (OPV optional)
15 months	MMR
18 months	DTP, OPV
2 years	HBPV
4-6 years	DTP, OPV
14-16 years	Td

Symbols:

DTP (diphtheria and tetanus toxoids with pertussis vaccine)

OPV (oral, attenuated poliovirus vaccine types 1, 2, and 3)

MMR (measles, mumps, and rubella vaccine)

HBPV (*Haemophilus* b polysaccharide vaccine)

Td (adult tetanus toxoid [full dose] and diphtheria toxoid [reduced dose] in combination)

32. *Gamma globulin or immunoglobulin*: This is an antibody preparation made from human plasma. For example, health officials may wish to give doses of immunoglobulin to children in a given day care center when cases of hepatitis appear.

33. *Impetigo*: Skin infection usually caused by the streptococcal bacteria. The lesions from this infection have several stages (vesicular, pustular and encrusted stages). The disease is usually acquired from other persons with impetigo, probably by direct contact. The incubation period of impetigo is not known.

34. *Incidence rate*: Refers to the number of cases of a disease over a defined period of time.

35. *Infection*: When an infectious agent multiplies in or on the body.

36. *Influenza*: This is an acute viral disease of the respiratory tract. Symptoms usually include fever, chills, headache, muscle aches, and sore throat. Man is the reservoir and other patients can be infected by airborne spread of contaminated droplets. The incubation period is short, usually 24 to 72 hours. A person may spread the disease up to 3 days from the onset. This disease is different from that caused by the organism *Haemophilus influenzae*, which is a bacterium.

37. *Mortality rate*: This term refers to the number of deaths due to a disease caused by an organism, divided by the number of persons infected.

38. *Meningococcus*: A bacterial organism with the name *Neisseria meningitidis*. It can cause meningitis.

39. *Meninges*: These are the tissues covering the brain. When they become infected and inflamed, the condition is called meningitis.

40. *Mycoplasma pneumoniae*: This bacterial organism can cause both upper and lower respiratory illness. The incidence of this disease is greatest during the fall and winter. The incubation period is 14 to 21 days.

41. *Otitis media*: Inflammation of the middle part of the ear. A very common infection. The organisms responsible for infection include *Streptococcus pneumoniae* and *Haemophilus influenzae*.

42. *Pediculosis*: Another word for lice. Mode of transmission is through direct contact with an infected person and indirectly by contact with his/her personal belongings. The incubation period is usually about 2 weeks.

43. *Prevalence*: This is the number of cases of a given disease in a population at risk during a given time period. For example, you may hear that the prevalence of asymptomatic *Giardia* in a day care center classroom on any given day might be 30 percent.

44. *Surveillance*: Systematic notation and evaluation of occurrence of disease. For example, state health departments may wish to do active surveillance for specific diseases, such as *Giardia* or *Haemophilus influenzae* in day care centers. Active surveillance means calling laboratories, day care centers, physicians and other day care health professionals to determine if disease is occurring. Passive surveillance is when one depends on volunteer reporting by health care personnel.

Disease	Communicable Period	Period of Incubation
1. Conjunctivitis	during the period of symptoms	24-72 hours
2. Hand, foot & mouth disease	acute stage of illness	3-5 days
3. Ringworm of the scalp	when lesions are present	10-14 days
4. Acute diarrhea	Depends on the actual organism. For bacterial organisms, it may be for several weeks. For common viral infections like Norwalk or rotavirus, it may be only a few days after onset of diarrhea.	Depends on the organism. For *Salmonella* it can be from 6-72 hours.
5. Diphtheria	approximately 2-4 weeks	2-5 days
6. Enterobiasis (Pinworms)	as long as eggs are present in the stool	4-6 weeks

7. Giardiasis	as long as the person is infected	
8. Hepatitis, type A	until the end of the incubation period; not usually after the onset of jaundice	15-50 days (usually around 30 days)
9. Measles	just before appearance of rash to 4 days after appearance of rash	10-14 days
10. Rubella (German measles)	from one week before to 4 days after appearance of rash	14-21 days
11. Erythema infectiosum (Fifth disease)	unknown	6-14 days
12. Salmonellosis	throughout the course of infection	6-72 hours
13. Scabies	until mites and eggs are destroyed (usually after 1-2 courses of therapy)	2-6 weeks in persons not previously exposed
14. Impetigo (due to staphylo-coccus)	as long as purulent lesions or the carrier state exists	unknown
15. Whooping cough	in untreated patients, from the onset of para-ysmal cough for 3 weeks	approximately 7-10 days

Adapted from:
MEDICAL TERMS FOR THE CHILD DAY CARE PROFESSIONAL AND CHILD DAY CARE TERMS FOR THE HEALTH PROFESSIONAL
Minnesota Department of Health
June, 1984

APPENDIX VIII

Additional Reading For The Health Consultant

1. Fein GG, Clarke-Stewart A: *Day Care in Context*, A Wiley Interscience Publication. New York, John Wiley and Sons, 1972
2. Ruopp R, O'Farrell B, Warner D, Rowe M, Freedman R: *A Day Care Guide for Administrators, Teachers, and Parents*. Cambridge, MA, The MIT Press, 1973
3. Provence S, Naylor A, Patterson J: *The Challenge of Daycare*. New Haven, Yale University Press, 1977
4. Highberger R, Schramna C: *Child Development for Day Care Workers*. Boston, Houghton-Mifflin Co, 1976
5. Robinson M, et al: *Who Will Mind the Babies?* National Center of Clinical Infant Programs (NCCIP), Washington, DC, 1984
6. Galensky E, Hooks W: *The New Extended Family: Day Care that Works*. Boston, Houghton-Mifflin, 1977
7. Ruopp R, Travers J, Glantz F, Coelon C: *Children at the Center*, in Nancy I, (ed): A Report of the National Day Care Study prepared by Abt Assoc, Inc, Cambridge, MA for Dept. of Health, Education, and Welfare, Washington, DC, 1979
8. *The Appropriateness of the Federal Interagency Day Care Requirements*. Report of Findings and Recommendations. Office of the Assistant Secretary for Planning and Evaluation, US Dept. of Health, Education, and Welfare, Washington, DC, 1978
9. Williams KA: *Childhood Emergency Sourcebook*. Available through Preschool Enrichment Team, Inc, 276 High St., Holyoke, MA 01040
10. Osterholm MT, Klein JO, Aronson SS, Pickering LK (Guest eds): Infectious Diseases in Child Day Care: Management and Prevention. Rev Infect Dis 1986;8:513-679

Index

First aid 90
  Instructions for day care programs 210-219
Floor, injury prevention 80
Floor space, requirement in physical setting 14
Fomite 223
Food preparation area 63-65
Food storage 24
  Site safety checklist 198-200
Formula, infant 65
Fracture 215
Frank Porter Graham Development Center 4

Gamma globulin 225
Garbage, storage and removal 62
Gender identification 17-18
German measles (rubella)
  Childhood immunization schedule 186-187
  Communicable and incubation period 227
  Staff immunization records 182-183
Giardia lamblia 223-224
Giardiasis 68, 224-225, 227
Gross motor play
  Injuries related to 76
  Planning of 77
Guidelines for Health Supervision 19
  Sample form 184-185
Guns, safety regulations 88-89

Haemophilus b polysaccharide vaccine (HBPV) 71, 186-187, 224-225
Haemophilus influenzae 222-226
Haemophilus influenzae type b 69, 71
  Childhood immunization schedule 186-187
  Vaccine for 71
Hair infection 69
Hallway safety checklist 196-197
Handicapped children 6, 32-39. *See also* disabled child
Hand washing, importance of 58-60
HBPV (*Haemophilus* b polysaccharide vaccine) 186-187, 224-225
Head injury 217
Head Start 4, 34, 116, 127
Health assessment form 138-139
Health care
  Policies 118-119
  As a scheduled activity 16
Health consultant 105-113
  Defining day care program 105